D0519684

Conflict and Health

Understanding Public Health series

Series editors: Nicki Thorogood and Ros Plowman, London School of Hygiene & Tropical Medicine (previous edition edited by Nick Black and Rosalind Raine)

Throughout the world, there is growing recognition of the importance of public health to sustainable, safe and healthy societies. The achievements of public health in nineteenth-century Europe were for much of the twentieth century overshadowed by advances in personal care, in particular in hospital care. Now, with the dawning of a new century, there is increasing understanding of the inevitable limits of individual health care and of the need to complement such services with effective public health strategies. Major improvements in people's health will come from controlling communicable diseases, eradicating environmental hazards, improving people's diets and enhancing the availability and quality of effective health care. To achieve this, every country needs a cadre of knowledgeable public health practitioners with social, political and organizational skills to lead and bring about changes at international, national and local levels.

This is one of a series of books that provides a foundation for those wishing to join in and contribute to the twenty-first-century regeneration of public health, helping to put the concerns and perspectives of public health at the heart of policy-making and service provision. While each book stands alone, together they provide a comprehensive account of the three main aims of public health: protecting the public from environmental hazards, improving the health of the public and ensuring high-quality health services are available to all. Some of the books focus on methods, others on key topics. They have been written by staff at the London School of Hygiene & Tropical Medicine with considerable experience of teaching public health to students from low-, middle- and high-income countries. Much of the material has been developed and tested with postgraduate students both in face-to-face teaching and through distance learning.

The books are designed for self-directed learning. Each chapter has explicit learning objectives, key terms are highlighted and the text contains many activities to enable the reader to test their own understanding of the ideas and material covered. Written in a clear and accessible style, the series will be essential reading for students taking postgraduate courses in public health and will also be of interest to public health practitioners and policy-makers.

Titles in the series

Analytical models for decision making: Colin Sanderson and Reinhold Gruen
Controlling communicable disease: Norman Noah
Conflict and Health: Natasha Howard, Egbert Sondorp and Annemarie ter Veen (eds)
Economic analysis for management and policy: Stephen Jan, Lilani Kumaranayake, Jenny Roberts, Kara Hanson and
     Kate Archibald
Economic evaluation: Julia Fox-Rushby and John Cairns (eds)
Environmental epidemiology: Paul Wilkinson (ed)
Environmental health policy: Megan Landon and Tony Fletcher
Financial management in health services: Reinhold Gruen and Anne Howarth
Global change and health: Kelley Lee and Jeff Collin (eds)
Health care evaluation: Sarah Smith, Don Sinclair, Rosalind Raine and Barnaby Reeves
Health promotion practice: Maggie Davies, Wendy Macdowall and Chris Bonell (eds)
Health promotion theory: Maggie Davies and Wendy Macdowall (eds)
Introduction to epidemiology, second edition: Ilona Carneiro and Natasha Howard
Introduction to health economics, second edition: Lorna Guinness and Virginia Wiseman (eds)
Issues in public health, second edition: Fiona Sim and Martin McKee (eds)
Making health policy, second edition: Kent Buse, Nicholas Mays and Gill Walt
Managing health services: Nick Goodwin, Reinhold Gruen and Valerie Iles
Medical anthropology: Robert Pool and Wenzel Geissler
Principles of social research: Judith Green and John Browne (eds)
Public health in history: Virginia Berridge, Martin Gorsky and Alex Mold
Sexual health: A public health perspective: Kaye Wellings, Kirstin Mitchell and Martine Collumbien
Understanding health services: Nick Black and Reinhold Gruen

Forthcoming titles:

Environments, health and sustainable development, second edition: Emma Hutchinson and Sari Kovats (eds)

Conflict and Health

Edited by Natasha Howard,
Egbert Sondorp and
Annemarie ter Veen

 Open University Press

Open University Press
McGraw-Hill Education
McGraw-Hill House
Shoppenhangers Road
Maidenhead
Berkshire
England
SL6 2QL

email: enquiries@openup.co.uk
world wide web: www.openup.co.uk

and Two Penn Plaza, New York, NY 10121-2289, USA

First published 2012

Copyright © London School of Hygiene & Tropical Medicine

All rights reserved. Except for the quotation of short passages for the purpose of criticism and review, no part of this publication may be reproduced, stored in a retrieval system, or transmitted, in any form or by any means, electronic, mechanical, photocopying, recording or otherwise, without the prior written permission of the publisher or a licence from the Copyright Licensing Agency Limited. Details of such licences (for reprographic reproduction) may be obtained from the Copyright Licensing Agency Ltd of Saffron House, 6–10 Kirby Street, London EC1N 8TS.

A catalogue record of this book is available from the British Library

ISBN-13: 978-0-33-524379-2 (pb)
ISBN-10: 0-33-524379-7 (pb)
eISBN: 978-0-33-524380-8

Library of Congress Cataloging-in-Publication Data
CIP data applied for

Typesetting and e-book compilations by
RefineCatch Limited, Bungay, Suffolk
Printed and bound by CPI Group (UK) Ltd, Croydon, CR0 4YY

Fictitious names of companies, products, people, characters and/or data that may be used herein (in case studies or in examples) are not intended to represent any real individual, company, product or event.

The *McGraw·Hill* Companies

"A much needed, eminently readable, concise and practical textbook ... New issues on humanitarian reform, non-communicable diseases, equity, corruption, and the role of military and private security firms are only some of the topics that have not been included in previous text books on this subject. I highly recommend this book for students and practitioners who wish to learn about the subject or simply update themselves on the latest developments in the field of conflict and public health."

Paul Spiegel, Deputy Director of the Division of Programme Support and Management at the United Nations High Commissioner for Refugees (UNHCR), Switzerland

"These are the most difficult environments to program in; physically, emotionally, politically and morally. Providing public health support and assistance here demands courage, rigor, a commitment to professionalism and an obsession with evidence. This book provides just such a foundation, equipping the student and practitioner to better understand the nature of conflict, the theory and practice of humanitarian assistance and the possibilities for recovery after conflict. It is destined to become an obligatory text for all humanitarian professionals."

Dr. Peter Walker, Irwin H. Rosenberg Professor of Nutrition and Human Security, Tufts University, USA

Dedicated to Alya Howard

Contents

List of Figures

List of Tables

List of authors

FIONA CAMPBELL is head of health policy for Merlin in Myanmar and has a background in nutrition, public heath, and development management. She has worked in development, in both advisory and programme management roles, and in the humanitarian sector with Merlin since 2006.

STEVE COMMINS is a lecturer at Luskin School of Public Affairs, University of California, Los Angeles, and strategy manager for fragile states at International Medical Corps (IMC). His work focuses on health and governance in fragile states and disaster risk reduction programmes.

SOPHIA CRAIG is a disaster and emergency management consultant who specializes in post-conflict humanitarian relief. She is a former Merlin country director and health cluster coordinator for the World Health Organization (WHO).

NADINE EZARD is a consultant with 19 years of experience with international non-governmental organizations (NGOs) and United Nations (UN) agencies, including 13 years in humanitarian health. With a background in clinical addiction medicine, she has skills across a range of areas of global public health and particular interest in building the evidence base for humanitarian intervention.

MICHELLE GAYER is an associate professor at the University of New South Wales and coordinator of Surge and Crisis support at WHO. Her work includes public health policy and planning in developing countries; emergency preparedness and response strategies; infectious disease epidemiology, risk assessment, surveillance, prevention and control in conflict and disaster; child health; vaccine-preventable disease and immunization; HIV, malaria and tuberculosis control.

PETER GIESEN is a strategic planning and monitoring and evaluation (M&E) consultant for humanitarian clients, including Médecins Sans Frontières (MSF), Red Cross national societies, IFRC, CARE, Simavi, Dutch Rehabilitation Consortium, Oxfam, UNICEF, and Netherlands HIV/AIDS consortium. He has worked for over 20 years in disaster response, monitoring and evaluation, and founded the Humanitarian Strategy in 2007 with the vision to deliver more useful and user-friendly monitoring and evaluation products.

ANDRÉ GRIEKSPOOR is a technical officer for policy, practice and evaluation in the Emergency Risk Management and Humanitarian Response Department, WHO. His responsibilities include health sector policy development in protracted crises and supporting post-crisis recovery planning processes. He has worked for WHO and MSF for over 10 years in countries such as South Sudan, Rwanda, Ethiopia, and Liberia.

RUKHSANA HAIDER is chairperson for the Training and Assistance for Health & Nutrition (TAHN) Foundation in Bangladesh and former regional advisor on nutrition for health and development for the WHO Southeast Asia Region. She currently works on nutrition in emergencies in Bangladesh.

LARA HO is health technical advisor for the International Rescue Committee's (IRC) program in DR Congo, focusing on post-conflict health system reconstruction. She previously worked for the IRC in Tanzania and Côte d'Ivoire in refugee and post-conflict settings.

MICHIEL HOFMAN is an advisor in operational strategy for MSF Belgium. Since 1993, he has worked for MSF in Liberia, DRC, Bosnia, Burundi, Sri Lanka, Brazil, South Sudan, Kosovo, Chechnya and Amsterdam, and as a freelance journalist between missions. In 2001, Michiel co-founded The Antares Foundation, a Dutch non-profit organization supporting local NGO provision of psychosocial support for staff in high-stress environments.

MAZEDA HOSSAIN is a lecturer in social epidemiology at the London School of Hygiene & Tropical Medicine (LSHTM). Her research focuses on gender-based violence among vulnerable populations in conflict-affected settings, women trafficked for sex, asylum seekers, migrant populations, and the design and evaluation of complex interventions

NATASHA HOWARD is a lecturer in global health and conflict at LSHTM. She has over 15 years of experience in health research and programme management in post-conflict and chronic emergencies, particularly in Myanmar and Afghanistan. Her research focuses on infectious disease control and social influences on health in conflict-affected settings, including violence and psychological resilience.

CHRIS LEWIS is a health advisor with the Department for International Development. He has previously worked with Save the Children, Tearfund and Medair, including work in fragile states and responses to natural disasters, outbreaks and conflict. His interests include primary health care, health systems strengthening and coordination, particularly in humanitarian settings.

ADRIANNA MURPHY is a PhD candidate in the European Centre on Health of Sociaties in Transition (ECOHOST) at LSHTM. Her research is in non-communicable diseases in low- and middle-income countries, currently specializing in social determinants of alcoholism in the former Soviet Union.

JAMES PALLETT is a clinical fellow in intensive care medicine at King's College Hospital, London. After obtaining membership of the Royal College of Surgeons of Edinburgh, James worked with MSF in the Central African Republic and as medical focal point for an emergency centre in Port-au-Prince, Haiti, in an area with high levels of gang-related conflict.

PREETI PATEL is a lecturer in global health and security at King's College London, teaching on complex political emergencies at the Department of War Studies and conflict and security at the Centre for Global Health. Her research interests include: capacity-building, governance and leadership issues in health systems of fragile states, tracking official development assistance for health in conflict-affected countries and global health initiatives.

VALERIE PERCIVAL is an assistant professor at the Norman Paterson School of International Affairs at Carleton University in Ottawa, Canada. Previously she worked as senior health advisor to the Canadian Department of Foreign Affairs and International Trade and was project director for the International Crisis Group in Kosovo.

PAUL SENDER is country director for Merlin in Myanmar. He trained in the UK in adult medicine, completed a higher specialist medical qualification in paediatrics, and has worked in medical and managerial positions for international NGOs, most recently in Myanmar and Afghanistan, for the past eight years.

EGBERT SONDORP is a senior advisor for health system strengthening at the Royal Tropical Institute (KIT) in Amsterdam and a senior lecturer in conflict and health at LSHTM.

ANNEMARIE TER VEEN is a senior advisor for health and education at KIT in Amsterdam. She has worked in humanitarian and post-conflict reconstruction in conflict-affected and post-conflict settings, including Afghanistan, Liberia, Rwanda and Somalia.

JEAN-FRANCOIS TRANI is an assistant professor at Brown School of Social Work, Washington University, St Louis. He has contributed to large-scale surveys on disability and vulnerability in Afghanistan, Sudan, Sierra Leone, Nepal and India.

PETER VENTEVOGE is a psychiatrist and medical anthropologist. He is affiliated with the dutch NGO Healthnet TPO, having worked with them as technical advisor for mental health in conflict-affected countries such as Afghanistan and Burundi. With the War Trauma Foundation he works as the Editor in-Chief of *Intervention, the international Journal of Mental Health, Psychosocial Work and Counselling in Areas of Armed Conflict.*

Acknowledgements

The editors are particularly grateful to the following colleagues for their generosity of time and intellectual rigour in reviewing chapters and sections:

- Section I – Anne Canavan, Sophia Craig, Tobias Denskus, Eiman Hussain, Anne Golaz, Elena Lucchi, Adrianna Murphy, and Emrys Shoemaker, and special thanks to Lara Ho for written contributions to Chapter 3;
- Section II – Karl Blanchet, Maria Kett, Besi Mpepo, James Pallet, Bayard Roberts, Claire Schofield, and Mesfin Teklu, and special thanks to Vickie Hawkins for written contributions to Chapter 7;
- Section III – Olga Bornemisza, Alya Howard, Eiman Hussain, Adrianna Murphy, Sridhar Venkatapuram, and special thanks to World Vision Canada for permitting use of the 2011 report *From Services to Systems: Entry Points for Donors and Non-state Partners Seeking to Strengthen Health Systems in Fragile States* as a partial basis for Chapter 13.

The editors wish to thank series editors Nicki Thorogood and Ros Plowman, and Alex Clabburn at McGraw-Hill Publishing. Open University Press and LSHTM have made every effort to obtain permission from copyright holders to reproduce material in this book and to acknowledge these sources correctly. Any omissions brought to our attention will be remedied in future editions.

Overview of the book

Introduction

This book is intended for self-directed learning and aims to provide the reader with an overview of current health-related challenges and policy debates about appropriate responses to populations affected by conflict. *Conflict* as used here refers to violent armed struggle between hostile groups, while *health* refers to the World Health Organization definition of complete physical, mental, and social well-being and not merely the absence of disease. Chapters will not usually distinguish between the three forms of organized political violence (i.e. state-based, non-state and one-sided) unless differences are relevant to the discussion.

The book is divided into three broad sections. The first section provides a theoretical overview of the nature and origins of conflict, the effects of conflict on society and population health, humanitarianism and the humanitarian system, including principles, aid and ethics. The second section covers practical approaches and issues in assessment, priority setting, health interventions, and quality assurance in conflict-affected settings. The final section describes approaches to reconstruction, including some of the complexities of the linkages between emergency relief and longer-term development, health system strengthening, health financing, and overarching policy themes.

Why study conflict and health?

There can be no development without security, and no security without development, and neither can be sustained without respect for human rights and the rule of law. (Kofi Annan)

The literature on conflict and health has increased substantially in the last decade. Substantial political theory and research on conflict and security support a relatively robust body of international human rights law. A wealth of humanitarian experience and guidance exists, addressing many operational questions in conflict settings. It is now possible, and therefore increasingly expected, to work as a humanitarian professional with a thorough grounding in both theory and practice.

Objectives of the book

After completing this book, you should be able to:

*   describe key political, economic and social factors that contribute to conflict and the effects of conflict on health;
*   identify institutional actors and approaches of the international humanitarian system;

- consider context-sensitive interventions for acute and chronic health care delivery and security;
- describe key issues and policy debates in the transition from relief to rehabilitation, health system strengthening, and post-conflict recovery.

Structure of the book

This book adapts the educational framework and content of the face-to-face *Conflict and Health* module taught at the London School of Hygiene & Tropical Medicine (LSHTM) for distance learning.

Section I (Chapters 1–5) introduces major theories of conflict, security and fragility. It considers direct and indirect effects of conflict on societies (e.g. displacement, death), the health burden of conflict, and the influence of human rights. Finally, it describes international responses, including aid architecture, the humanitarian system, military and security agencies, and the role of the media.

Section II (Chapters 6–11) focuses on practical aspects of humanitarian intervention. Topics include assessment and priority setting, health service delivery in difficult settings, interventions to reduce disease and improve health, monitoring and evaluation, and security and protection.

Section III (Chapters 12–14) outlines reconstruction issues during and post-conflict. Topics include early recovery, health reform, health system strengthening, financing and delivery models, and policy issues.

Each chapter includes:

- an overview;
- learning outcomes;
- self-study activities;
- concluding summary;
- feedback on activities.

Words in the glossary appear in **bold** at the first mention.

Guidance for activities

We recommend that you attempt the activities as they appear in the text, and refer back to the preceding explanatory text if you find a question unclear or difficult. You should complete the whole of each activity before reading the relevant feedback, as this will help you assess your understanding of the material presented. Any required mathematical skills will be basic.

SECTION I

Context

Causes of conflict

Preeti Patel

Overview

The aim of this chapter is to provide an overview of some contemporary explanatory theories of the causes of conflict within societies. Concepts from war studies literature and research are used to examine competing explanations and potential contributing factors in relation to civil conflicts since the end of the Cold War in 1991.

Learning outcomes

When you have completed this chapter, you should be able to:

- describe the changing nature of contemporary armed conflict
- summarize the most influential explanatory theories on the causes of conflict
- review current debates on the causes of conflict

Changing nature of conflict

Since the early 1990s, many more civil conflicts (sometimes called intra-state conflicts, as they usually take place within national borders) than **international conflicts** (i.e. conflicts between countries) have occurred. While there are many in-depth theories on the causes of conflicts in individual countries, this chapter will summarize the most influential general theories of conflict.

The nature of armed conflict appears to have changed since the end of the Cold War, in what is described as a shift from **old wars** to **new wars**. Mark Duffield argues that new wars can also be called 'network wars' or 'complex political emergencies' by those in the humanitarian sector, as these conflicts tend to cut through state territories and are linked to global financial and criminal networks. Essentially, new wars comprise a new form of privatized non-territorial network consisting of **state** and non-state actors working beyond the competence of territorially defined governments (Duffield, 2001).

New wars have a strong global dimension. Based on qualitative research in Bosnia-Herzegovina and elsewhere, Mary Kaldor argues that a new type of organized violence (i.e. violence for private gain) emerged in the 1980s and early 1990s, which can be described as new war. What is new about 'new wars' can be understood in the context of the weakening of national sovereignty through globalization. Kaldor argues that new wars are increasingly intertwined with other global risks such as the spread of **disease, vulnerability** to natural disasters, poverty and homelessness (Kaldor, 2007). Globalization contributes to conflict when production collapses and armed forces and/ or rebel organizations are sustained via remittances, diaspora fund-raising, external government assistance, and the diversion of international humanitarian aid. For example, during the recent conflict in Somalia, a United Nations report claimed that up to half of food aid – valued at approximately $485 million in 2009 – was being diverted through contractors, World Food Programme (WFP) staff and local armed groups (Bailey, 2010). In new wars, the distinction between war and organized crime is blurred (Kaldor, 2007). New wars generate an economy based on plunder, or violent theft of goods. For example, resource plunder has been driving the conflict in the Democratic Republic of Congo in recent years.

Proponents of the new war hypothesis argue that contemporary wars are distinct from old wars in their methods of warfare, their causes and their financing (Di John, 2008). Old wars tended to involve ideological conflicts between nations, were fought by armed forces in uniform, and decisive encounters were on the battlefield (Kaldor, 1999). Old wars were fought according to certain rules, at least in theory, that were critical to establishing the legitimacy of wars. These rules were codified in the late nineteenth and early twentieth centuries in the Geneva and Hague Conventions, which were concerned with minimizing civilian casualties and treating prisoners of war humanely (Kaldor, 2007). New war proponents claim that battles are rare in contemporary wars, and significant violence and human rights violations are directed against civilians (Kaldor, 2007). A common feature of new wars is population expulsion, resulting in large numbers of refugees and internally displaced persons. New wars are very difficult to end, as various warring factions have vested interests in continuing violence for ethnic, economic and political motives – hence the term **protracted conflict** has been used to describe many long-term conflicts such as in Afghanistan, Myanmar, and Somalia.

The new war hypothesis can be criticized as lacking empiricism, as many of the features described above are not particularly new. Violence targeted at civilians, widespread criminality, identity or ethnic politics, the presence of non-state actors and human rights violations have been present in many past conflicts. Each conflict has unique contextual features, but theoretical models such as the new war hypothesis can provide a foundation for comparative analysis and interpretation of conflict.

Explanatory theories of conflict

Ethnicity and identity

Significant attention has been devoted to the role of **ethnicity** and ethnic tensions as a cause of conflict and a key feature of new wars. Recent examples include Rwanda, Burundi and the Balkan wars. **Ethnic conflicts** refer to wars between ethnic groups or in which ethnic difference is central to the conflict (Smith, 2004). This includes identity conflict where warring groups claim power because of a particular identity, such as clan (e.g. Somalia), religion (e.g. Nigeria, the Philippines) or language (e.g. Namibia).

The two main theoretical discourses on ethnic or cultural conflict are (i) primordial and (ii) manufactured/invented theory. Primordial social theory suggests that ethnic conflict is rooted in ancient group hatreds and loyalties and that these old sources of enmity and memories of past atrocities make violence hard to avoid (Kaplan, 1994). Paul Collier found that ethnic dominance is an influential factor in the trajectory of civil conflict. Ethnic dominance occurs in countries in which the largest single ethnic group is approximately 45–90% of the population (Collier, 2000). Manufactured ethnic conflict theory suggests that ethnicity is an instrument of mobilization for political leaders.

Political leaders may deliberately 'rework historical memories' to strengthen identity in the competition for power and resources (Stewart, 2002). For example, the post-election violence resulting from contested 2007 elections in Kenya was worsened by manufactured ethnic civil unrest (Stewart, 2002).

Contemporary wars construct new sectarian identities (e.g. religious, ethnic, tribal) that undermine a sense of shared political community. Kaldor argues that a purpose of new wars is to recreate a sense of political community along new divisive lines through the manufacture of fear and hate. A key factor driving ordinary people to participate in ethnic conflict is fear. For example, before and during the Rwandan genocide in 1994, Hutus were subjected to a major propaganda campaign suggesting Tutsis and the Rwandan Patriotic Front were planning to kill them (Keen, 2008).

Politics and economics

David Keen, Francis Stewart, and other critics of ethnic theories of conflict argue that the ancient hatreds analysis is too mono-causal and ignores political and economic roots of conflict (Stewart, 2002). These critics argue that even in armed conflicts involving parties divided by ethnicity, the situation cannot be analysed adequately by looking at ethnicity alone. Gurr's research on relative deprivation in societies and its association with conflict suggests that if there is significant discrepancy between what people think they deserve and what they think they will get (i.e. relative deprivation), there is a likelihood of conflict or rebellion (Gurr, 1970). Political violence is considered more likely if people think that the current leadership or socioeconomic/political system is illegitimate (Gurr, 1970). This perspective has some currency in explaining recent conflicts in North Africa and the Middle East. Scholars such as Mamdani have argued that colonial legacies shaped institutions and ethnic identities, laying the foundations for conflict in many countries (Mamdani, 1996).

Research by Collier, Cramer, and Keen indicates the importance of economic conditions and the political system (Collier, 2008). During the last decade, a group of economists working with the World Bank conducted statistical analyses on the causes of **civil war**. Findings have been reported in international reports on security and development, including the 2011 World Development Report on *Conflict, Security and Development*, and played a prominent role in influencing conflict resolution and management strategies within several international organizations (World Bank, 2011).

Collier and Hoeffler, of Oxford University, developed econometric models based on several economic, political and social **risk factors**, to predict the outbreak of civil conflict globally based on empirical patterns over the period 1960–1999 (Collier and Hoeffler, 2004). Their findings indicated that the risk of civil conflict was systematically related to selected economic conditions, including dependence on primary commodity exports and low national income, while social **grievances** such as inequality, lack of democracy, and ethnic and religious division within society had little effect on the risk of conflict (Collier, 2000).

Political science explains conflict in terms of motive (e.g. a rebellion occurs when grievances are sufficiently acute that people want to engage in violent protest). Grievances may include political repression, inequality, injustice, or religious and ethnic divisions. Civil war thus occurs as an intense political contest, fuelled by grievances so severe that they were not addressed by peaceful methods of political protest. Collier argues that contemporary conflicts are driven overwhelmingly by 'greed' rather than 'grievance', that is, grievances and hatreds do not cause conflict; rather economic issues such as dependence on primary commodity exports, low average incomes, slow economic growth and large diasporas are more significant and powerful explanations of the causes of civil war (Collier, 2000). Collier and colleagues also argue that civil wars occur where rebel organizations were financially viable – conflict will occur where it is possible, regardless of motivation (Collier et al., 2009).

This interpretation of resource–conflict links led Collier and colleagues to formulate the *greed and grievance model*, which hypothesizes a combination of **greed** and grievance causing and fuelling civil conflicts. Thus, the question became not which cause was more important, but rather how the different causes interact (e.g. whose greed and whose grievance, or how do the greedy manipulate the grievances of others in society?).

Activity 1.1

Select a conflict-affected country that you find interesting. Do you think the greed and grievance hypothesis is useful and relevant in your chosen country? What alternative causes of conflict can you list for your chosen country?

Collier's conflict risk analysis

Researchers have proposed a number of interrelated risk factors causing and/or fuelling conflict. These were drawn together in Collier's risk analysis and include natural resources (e.g. **resource curse**) and primary commodity exports, poverty, youth unemployment, militarization, ethnic dominance, diaspora, regime instability, geography, history, and regional conflict.

The resource curse argument, suggesting abundant natural resources (e.g. diamonds, oil) are often associated with greater incidence, intensity and duration of civil conflict, is one of the most influential explanations of contemporary conflict (Di John, 2008). Collier's early research indicated that the most powerful factor for a country's risk of developing civil war is heavy dependence on primary commodity exports such as oil or diamonds (Collier, 2000). Primary commodity exports are particularly vulnerable to looting as their production relies on assets that are immobile and lasting. 'The same characteristics that make it easy for governments to tax them, make it easy for rebels to loot them' (Collier, 2000). Resources such as alluvial diamonds and narcotics can be extracted and transported by individuals or small groups of unskilled workers (Ballentine and Nitzchke, 2003). These resources provide direct rents for rebels and income for local communities, making wartime exploitation so profitable that combatants could prefer protracted war to peace. Examples of conflicts centred on natural resource extortion include diamonds in Sierra Leone, cocaine in Colombia, and timber in Cambodia.

Poverty or slow economic growth is an important risk factor for civil conflict. Collier found that the odds a civil war will occur in a low-income country were 15 times higher than in a high-income country, while a doubling of per-capita income could halve the risk of civil war. The risk of conflict may be higher in low-income countries as the poorest people may feel they have little to lose from joining a rebel group, making rebel recruitment relatively cheap and easy. Laurent Kabila, former president and rebel leader in the Democratic Republic of Congo, claimed that organizing and leading a rebellion in what was Zaire was easy – 'all you needed was $10,000 and a satellite phone' (Collier, 2008).

Youth unemployment, particularly among males, relates to poverty and can critically influence the probability of violent conflict. Boys and young men can be pushed to join the military in low-income countries with minimal economic and educational opportunities and rapid population growth (e.g. Angola, Sierra Leone). Lack of jobs and opportunities creates frustration and can make children and unemployed youth prime candidates for recruitment as child soldiers. Both criminality and rebellion rely heavily on this disfranchised segment of the population. In Sierra Leone, for example, the Revolutionary United Forces recruited young male drug addicts, controlling them by drug supplies.

Militarization and the proliferation of arms can encourage economic violence, as can high defence spending, the availability of arms, and the presence of armed non-state actors. The Balkans and the Horn of Africa are examples of regions where availability of arms and presence of non-state actors increased the risk of conflicts.

The concept of ethnic dominance, as noted above, is influential though contested as a risk factor in the trajectory of civil conflict. Proponents cite examples of clashes between Hutus and Tutsis in Rwanda and Burundi and between Sunnis, Shiites, and Kurds in Iraq (Collier, 2008). Conversely, societies that are ethnically and religiously diverse are seen as having less risk of conflict (Collier, 2000).

Larger diasporas are associated with risk of civil conflict. Diasporas can be an important source of finance for rebel groups, and Collier argues they sometimes hold romanticized attachments to their group of origin or nurse grievances as a form of asserting continued belonging (Collier, 2000). Diaspora populations tend to be wealthier than populations in their country of origin and can afford to finance a conflict. And they do not have to bear the direct consequences of the conflict. Examples of diasporas financing conflict include US Tamil and Irish communities in the United States supporting the Tamil Tigers in Sri Lanka and Irish Republican Army activities in Northern Ireland, respectively.

Regime instability is considered important, as established democracies and autocracies appear less prone to conflict. Pinker argues that the rise of the nation state and the spread of democracy are among factors linked to a decline of conflict and violence (Pinker, 2011). Conversely, the transition between one form of rule and another is associated with higher risk of conflict. The recent political conflicts in North Africa and the Middle East are examples of transition from one form of governance to another.

Geography is clearly important. Large countries with dispersed populations, such as the Democratic Republic of Congo, are challenging for security and governance. Countries with large areas of mountainous terrain, such as Nepal and Afghanistan, pose challenges for security forces as rebel organizations can find suitable places to form and hide (Collier, 2008).

The history of conflict is important, as countries that have experienced violent conflict in the past ten years have a very high chance of recurrence. This may be because the same structural factors that initially predisposed conflict often continue and mobilizing people through group memories is more effective with a history of conflict. Examples include Afghanistan, Somalia and Indonesia.

Regional conflicts are likely to affect conflict risk among neighbouring territories, particularly due to the flow of refugees, arms, and illicit goods. Examples include the Horn of Africa and the Balkans. In Kosovo, conflicts in neighbouring states and the spill-over effects they generated significantly altered the political economy of the crisis from one of peaceful resistance to violent conflict (Ballentine and Nitzchke, 2003).

Criticism of Collier's conflict risk analysis

Criticism of Collier's analysis and methodology falls into five main categories: (i) data reliability, (ii) categorization index reliability, (iii) mono-causal reliance, (iv) mono-dimensional analysis, and (v) domestic focus.

First, country-level data from **conflict-affected** countries can be unreliable (Cramer, 2006). Christopher Cramer argues that geographic variables such as natural resources, population distribution, ethnic composition and terrain can contain poor approximations of sub-national variations, which is problematic as most civil wars are geographically limited to small parts of a country (Buhaug and Lujala, 2004).

Second, the ethno-linguistic fragmentation index Collier used might be inaccurate. For example, while it might be possible to differentiate Hutus from Tutsis through an identity card in Rwanda, this is not the case in every conflict-affected country with different ethnic groups.

The third category of criticism is reliance on greed as a motivator. Cramer argues that lootable mineral resources are not the initial cause of civil wars, but rents can help conflicts to persist as the means of finance become a source of profit. Laurie Nathan is critical of Collier's interpreting his main risk factor, dependence on primary commodities, as greed-related. Instead, Nathan argues primary commodity exports could be linked to grievance in association with poor public service provision, corruption, and mismanagement and perhaps more indicative of poor governance than the availability of financial opportunities for rebellion (Nathan, 2005). Nathan argues that political variables such as repression and discrimination are not easily quantifiable and other factors relevant to the causes of civil war, such as history, ideology, propaganda, leadership and ethnic politics, cannot be quantified meaningfully (Nathan, 2005).

Fourth, Collier's analysis is mono-dimensional, as rebels are treated as homogeneous and government virtually ignored. Nathan criticizes Collier's work for not sufficiently analysing rebel behaviour and patterns, as the model does not stratify rebels involved, where they come from, or what motivates them beyond financial aspects in Collier's greed analysis (Nathan, 2005; Cramer, 2006). Crucially, Nathan and Keen argue that Collier's model ignores the role of government as a decision-maker or international actor, focusing almost entirely on the decisions, actions, and motives of rebels (Keen, 2008). While Collier's model covers the country's political system and degree of freedom or repression, which reflects government character, it does not consider the kinds of governmental decision, action, and motive that contribute to civil war. For example, outbreaks of conflict in the Democratic Republic of Congo and Sierra Leone were preceded by decades of political misrule and corruption by a parastatal elite, which exacerbated economic deterioration and institutional decay in both countries, ultimately resulting in state collapse (Ballentine and Nitzchke, 2003). Before and during the conflict, government soldiers in Sierra Leone were observed attacking civilians, engaging in illegal diamond mining, dressing as rebels and selling arms to rebels. A key weakness in the analysis of the Sierra Leonean conflict was the overwhelming focus on rebel abuses, while government corruption and solders' abuses were virtually unaddressed (Keen, 2008).

Fifth, Collier's focus was almost entirely domestic. Nathan, Keen and others note that Collier's model does not sufficiently consider regional and international factors, which are part of the structural context or influence in terms of rebels' decisions (the main exceptions being regional conflicts and the affected country's diaspora).

Academics and policy-makers argue that 'civil war' is not an accurate descriptor for most contemporary conflicts, as key actors and conflicts are generally not confined to national boundaries, instead tending to have strong regional and global dimensions

(Ballentine and Nitzchke, 2003). Regional and global factors include: predatory involvement of neighbouring countries, global criminal gangs involved in illicit arms trading, narcotics and commodities, private security firms and mercenaries, global multinational companies, and diasporas. Examples of regional and global influence include the prominent role played by the United States in the Iraq and Afghanistan wars, Ethiopia in Somalia, and China's support of the Sudanese regime through oil purchases and arms sales and of President Mugabe's regime in Zimbabwe through military equipment sales (Keen, 2008). Regional and national actors and dynamics significantly influence the character and duration of conflict and can also complicate the conflict resolution process and **post-conflict** stability by increasing the number of potential conflict profiteers (Ballentine and Nitzchke, 2003).

Activity 1.2

Choose a conflict-affected country and list how many of Collier's conflict risk factors might apply to your chosen country.

Structural determinants of conflict

Structural determinants of conflict are useful for understanding that explanations of violent armed conflict are normally multi-dimensional (Galtung, 1969). This section summarizes three current hypotheses: (i) horizontal inequalities, (ii) social contract, and (iii) green wars.

Horizontal inequalities

Frances Stewart proposed that what she termed 'horizontal inequalities' (i.e. inequalities in economic and political resources between culturally defined groups) contribute to the causes of conflict (Stewart, 2002). She suggests that culture, religion, geography and social class may divide groups, but these group differences only result in conflict when there are also differences in relation to the distribution and exercise of political and economic power. In such situations, relatively deprived groups are likely to seek redress or be persuaded by their leaders to do so. Relatively privileged groups may resort to conflict to protect their privileges when they think these might be threatened.

The horizontal inequalities hypothesis is persuasive in some cases – Angola's protracted civil war began as an anti-colonial struggle and only later did natural resource exploitation became the dominant source of belligerent funding for both rebels and government. In Sierra Leone, horizontal inequalities were visible in endemic unemployment and lack of access to education among youth (Ballentine and Nitzchke, 2003). In Nepal, grievances over systemic socioeconomic exclusion and widespread poverty provided impetus for conflict (Ballentine and Nitzchke, 2003).

Failure of social contract

The failure of **social contract** may contribute to conflict. The hypothesis that social stability is based on a hypothetical contract between people and state, in which people accept state authority while the government provides services (e.g. security, health, education, sanitation) and reasonable economic conditions (e.g. employment), has Classical roots (Pettit, 1997). Worsening economic conditions result in worsening state services in many low- and middle-income countries, which can lead to a breakdown in social contract and sometimes to conflict (Stewart, 2002). David Keen's research describes the role of international financial institutions (e.g. International Monetary Fund, World Bank) in fuelling conflict in Sierra Leone by encouraging inflation, major devaluation, and creation of private oligopolies when state enterprises were privatized. These liberalization policies were associated with a massive reduction of state services, including health and education, which fuelled grievances (Keen, 2008).

Green war hypothesis

A **green war hypothesis** argues that environmental degradation can increase poverty and insecurity, thus contributing to the likelihood of conflict (Homer-Dixon, 2001). Thomas Homer-Dixon argues that rapid increases in population will increase demand for natural resources, leading to scarcity of renewable resources such as arable land, water, and forests. Environmental scarcities are expected by many to have profound social consequences, which could lead to ethnic clashes, insurrections, urban violence, and other forms of conflict, particularly in low- and middle-income countries. Homer-Dixon bases his hypothesis on research on water shortages in China, population growth in sub-Saharan Africa, and land distribution in Mexico. Homer-Dixon argues that unequal distribution of resources can lead to conflict over resource scarcity, but is careful to point out that the effects of environmental scarcity are indirect and act in combination with other social, political and economic grievances (Homer-Dixon, 2001). Leading theories on causes of conflict generally describe ecological risks as peripheral, in that they may accelerate or exacerbate a conflict but are not usually seen as the root cause.

Current research does not suggest that climate change will drive conflict, except where rapidly deteriorating water resources cut across existing tensions, weak institutions, and weak governance (World Bank, 2011). Interlinked challenges such as changing patterns of energy consumption, scarce and non-renewable resources, and increasing demand for food imports relying on land, water and energy, will undoubtedly increase the pressure on low- and middle-income and fragile states (World Bank, 2011).

Just as there is almost never a single, identifiable root cause of war, it is difficult to prove a direct causal link between environmental change and conflict (Sondorp and Patel, 2003). Academics and most policy-makers agree that further evidence is necessary to determine the impact of global environmental change on land availability, food prices and weather, each of which can affect conflict vulnerability.

Conclusions

This chapter outlines the changing nature of conflict, the new war hypothesis, influential explanatory theories on causes of conflict, the role of inequality within countries, and the green war hypothesis. No general explanatory model will capture all aspects of the causes of a phenomenon as complex as war (Nathan, 2005). Conflict is clearly multi-causal and the causes that fuel a conflict may be different from the root causes that initiated it. The studies and explanatory models described in this chapter identify factors likely to predispose groups to conflict. It is important to analyse the unique context and causes of conflict for each conflict-affected country, considering relevant historical, ethnic, social, economic, and political factors, as well as the regional and international dimensions of that conflict. However, an understanding of general theories on causes of conflict is necessary for peace-building and conflict-prevention activities. The next chapter discusses the effects of conflict on societies.

Feedback on activities

Feedback on Activity 1.1

The causes of conflict tend to be context-specific. There may be greed-related resource abundance factors that relate to Collier's work. There may also be greed factors linked to environmental scarcity such as water or land shortages. Environmental insecurity or unjust resource exploitation also may be related to political factors. Overall, there tends to be a range of both greed- and grievance-related risk factors in most conflict-affected countries.

Feedback on Activity 1.2

The causes of conflict tend to be context-specific and whether Collier's risk factors apply to your chosen country will depend on a number of multi-causal overlapping factors. These may be political and/or institutional factors such as power struggles between elites, political exclusion and marginalization of certain groups or individuals. Other political factors such as legitimacy of political leaders, corruption, identity or ethnic politics could also be relevant for your chosen country. There may be socioeconomic factors such as a breakdown in the social contract, inequality and poverty that may also be relevant for your chosen country. There may be greed-related resource abundance factors that are closely related to Collier's work. There may also be greed factors linked to environmental scarcity such as water or land shortages. Environmental insecurity or unjust resource exploitation may also be related to political factors. Overall, there tends to be a range of both greed- and grievance-related risk factors in most conflict-affected countries.

2 Effects of conflict on societies

Sophia Craig

Overview

The aim of this chapter is to provide an overview of the effects of conflict on societies, focusing on population displacement and basic needs. Concepts from humanitarian literature and fieldwork in conflict and post-conflict settings are used to examine the societal effects of conflict.

Learning outcomes

When you have completed this chapter, you should be able to:

- describe the effects of conflict on human development
- explain the relationship between vulnerability and resilience and ways in which conflict affects vulnerable groups
- identify challenges to basic needs faced by conflict-affected populations

Effects of conflict on human development

The **cost of conflict** is determined by subtracting current welfare in a country from the expected welfare the country should have achieved in the absence of conflict (Bozzoli et al., 2010). An effective measure of conflict's true costs should include both direct (e.g. injury, death, human rights abuses, psychological disorders) and indirect effects (e.g. mortality and morbidity resulting from population displacement, infrastructure destruction, lack of food, lack of health care, environmental degradation).

Direct effects of conflict are typically attributable to combat-related deaths and injuries, while **indirect effects** are those that are not directly attributable to a physical or weapons attack but rather due to a combination of factors that often continue into the post-conflict period. Although young males generally suffer most from the direct effects of conflict (e.g. death and injury from fighting), women and children suffer disproportionately from indirect effects, including displacement, disease, and **malnutrition** (World Bank, 2004). The indirect effects of conflict can be devastating at a societal level. Conflict can destroy economic infrastructure, damage the local ecosystem, restrict communications, lower investment, and restrict export markets and foreign exchange earnings. Economic activities are disrupted, while increased military spending results in reduced funding for social services.

The World Bank states that in countries affected by violent conflict, poverty reduction is slower than in peaceful countries (World Bank, 2004). For countries recovering from protracted conflict, the effects are more devastating and long lasting. After a civil war it takes an average of 14 years of peace to regain original growth paths (World Bank, 2004). The erosion of public institutions and services such as water, sanitation, shelter, food and health limits human development and places the lives of the most vulnerable at risk. Most child illness, injury and death occurs in the months and years after a conflict has ceased.

In conflict-affected and **fragile states**, people are more than twice as likely to see their children die before age 5 and more than three times as likely to be unable to send their children to school (World Bank, 2004). Key infrastructure (e.g. hospitals, schools, factories, roads, communications, water treatment) is often destroyed and essential services disrupted. Farming and food production may be damaged or disrupted due to fighting, population displacement, broken supply chain or environmental degradation. Families may be separated by displacement. People may lose their livelihoods and possessions. Institutions are also vulnerable to conflict. Hospitals, which are reliant on both an efficient supply chain (e.g. pharmaceuticals, medical supplies) and staff (e.g. doctors, nurses, support staff) will be particularly vulnerable to the disruptive effects of conflict.

Conflict can compromise society's ability to protect its population, resulting in increased violence, **morbidity** and **mortality**. This lawlessness, when individuals and government are no longer regulated by laws but by arbitrary actions, is described as a breakdown of the **rule of law**. A state governed by the rule of law provides its citizens with order: predictable and efficient rulings, equality before the law, and human rights (Belton, 2009). When a breakdown of the rule of law occurs, key governance institutions and services (e.g. functioning judicial system, constitutional laws, law enforcement agencies) are disrupted or destroyed. The absence of the rule of law encourages illicit activities for both control (e.g. the use of sexual violence during civil wars in Liberia and Peru) and profit (e.g. human trafficking, drug smuggling, looting).

A breakdown in the rule of law encourages corruption during and after conflict. The World Bank (2004) estimates the global cost of corruption at $1 trillion, while development aid totals approximately $100 billion. Corruption can include bribery, embezzlement, nepotism, cronyism and fraud. Often countries plagued by high levels of corruption are more vulnerable to conflict, and conflict-affected countries are vulnerable to corruption.

In conflict-affected countries, humanitarian programming can be derailed by corruption. It can result in misallocation of resources intended to alleviate suffering and further increases the vulnerability of conflict-affected populations. Corruption reduces net income among poor and middle-income groups and decreases access to basic needs such as food, health care and education. Corruption also erodes confidence in government, creating unrest and distrust that could further destabilize a fragile peace. According to Transparency International's *Corruption Perceptions Index* (CPI), which measures domestic and public sector corruption, unstable governments with legacies of conflict tend to be the most corrupt. In 2011, for example, Afghanistan, Myanmar, Somalia, and North Korea were ranked by the CPI as the most corrupt countries in the world.

Measuring the effects of conflict

Given the complex effect of conflict on societies, measurement can be difficult. Economic assessments of conflict often focus on how the gross domestic product (GDP) of a country has been affected. Economic costing initiatives suggest that average economic output is reduced by approximately 1–3% each year that a country experiences conflict (Bozzoli et al., 2010). GDP in neighbouring countries is also affected, with neighbours suffering approximately one-third of the losses experienced by

countries in conflict (Bozzoli et al., 2010). Proponents of economic methods of measuring conflict suggest that income mirrors and integrates the progression of other
measures of human development, such as health outcomes and access to education
(Bozzoli et al., 2010). While economic assessments have the advantage of being straightforward in their use of standard indices and provision of quantifiable measures, they
cannot easily account for other costs of conflict (e.g. psychological, social, cultural,
environmental). Other composite indices, such as the *Human Development Index* (HDI),
have been proposed instead. Figure 2.1 shows World Bank estimates of the poverty gap
between conflict-affected and unaffected countries in recent decades.

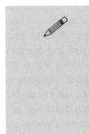

Activity 2.1

A country has experienced a protracted conflict for 15 years, devastating its
infrastructure, economy and social structures. It is now ranked near the bottom of
the HDI. Although a peace deal was negotiated, there are concerns that the country
could relapse into conflict.
2.1.1 Explain how you might assess the cost of conflict to this country.
2.1.2 List the types of problems a country with a low HDI ranking might experience.

Vulnerability and resilience

Vulnerability and resilience theory

Vulnerability and resilience are complex, interrelated concepts used in several disci-
plines (e.g. psychology, sociology, development, security, risk management). The more

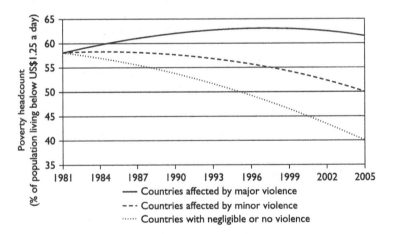

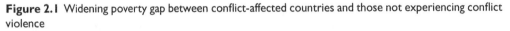

Figure 2.1 Widening poverty gap between conflict-affected countries and those not experiencing conflict
violence

Source: World Bank (2011).

vulnerable a person or community is, the less resilient to the harmful effects of conflict. **Social vulnerability** refers to the susceptibility of individuals, groups and societies to the adverse effects of shocks and multiple stressors to which they are exposed (e.g. abuse, social exclusion, disaster, conflict). A commonly accepted definition of vulnerability, from the International Strategy for Disaster Risk Reduction, is 'the conditions determined by physical, social, economic, and environmental factors or processes, which increase the susceptibility of a community to the impact of hazards' (UNISDR, 2004: 16).

Two influential models of social vulnerability, *risk-hazard* (RH) and *pressure and release* (PAR), have been adapted with variable success to analysing vulnerability in conflict settings. The more popular PAR model describes disaster or conflict as the intersection of those processes generating vulnerability with those generating hazards. Vulnerability can thus be considered in three progressive levels of root causes (e.g. weak governance, lack of access to political power and resources) creating dynamic pressures (i.e. processes that transform root causes into unsafe conditions, e.g. rapid urbanization, deforestation) that lead to unsafe conditions (e.g. violence, forced displacement) (Wisner et al., 2004).

The concept of **resilience** is closely related to vulnerability, but focuses on individual and group strengths rather than deficits. Resilience refers to the capacity of an individual or community to absorb shocks and adjust to changes while retaining essential stability and identity. Thus, a resilience framework focuses not on correcting deficits, but on promoting a social environment conducive to individual and group well-being. Types of resilience include psychological (i.e. individual), social (e.g. family, community), institutional, economic and ecological (Cutter et al., 2008). For the purpose of this chapter, we can think of social resilience as the ability of families and communities to adapt to and recover from the effects of conflict.

Vulnerable groups

Although conflict increases risk for all members of society, it is usually the politically, socially and economically marginalized groups of society that are most vulnerable to the effects of conflict (World Bank, 2011). Research indicates that conflict often exacerbates social inequities and widens the gap between rich and poor (World Bank, 2011). Social structures present before a conflict (e.g. wealth, law, religion, class, **gender**, ethnicity) generally determine who will be at greatest risk during conflict. According to the United Nations Food and Agriculture Organization (FAO), **vulnerable groups** are vulnerable under any circumstances (e.g. adults cannot provide adequately for the household due to **disability** or age). Factors determining vulnerability include socioeconomic (e.g. employment, income, housing), human assets (e.g. access to education and health care), and social assets (e.g. solidarity networks, reciprocal relations between households, relations with government and private institutions). Vulnerable groups can include displaced populations, children, elderly or disabled people, and those suffering from acute or chronic diseases (e.g. AIDS).

In assessing vulnerable population groups, consider physical and socioeconomic vulnerabilities and contextual effects of conflict specific to that group. For example, women are not designated as a vulnerable group during conflict, rather states are required to recognize their equal rights under the 1979 Convention on the Elimination of All Forms of Discrimination against Women. **International humanitarian law** (IHL), including Articles 76–77 of Protocol I additional to the 1977 Geneva Conventions, recognizes children as vulnerable and that women can be vulnerable in some circumstances (e.g. pregnancy, childbirth). In societies where women experience socioeconomic and political marginalization, conflict can result in increased human rights abuses, poverty, and victimization. Increased vulnerability can result in establishment or increase of human trafficking, sex work, intimate-partner violence, rape, **honour killing** and suicide (Handrahan, 2004). The International Committee of the Red Cross (ICRC) notes:

> in some conflicts, when women, as the bearers of future generations, are considered to be the depositories of cultural and ethnic identity, they may be vulnerable to attacks or threats from within the community if they do not conform to their assigned role. They may also be targeted by the enemy with a view to changing or destroying this role. The use of sexual violence as a method of warfare and the requirement that women bear more children to replace sons that have died make women especially vulnerable. (ICRC, 2007)

Although women are often considered vulnerable during conflict, many show remarkable resilience as combatants or by assuming responsibility for their families in exceptionally challenging circumstances. Table 2.1 shows gender-disaggregated effects of conflict.

Table 2.1 Gender-disaggregated effects of conflict on individuals and communities

	Direct effects	Indirect effects
Men	Higher rates of morbidity and mortality from battle deaths	Risk of ex-combatants' involvement in criminal or illegal activities and difficulties in finding livelihoods
	Higher likelihood to be detained or missing	Increased prevalence of other forms of violence – particularly domestic violence
	Sexual and gender-based violence: sex-selective massacres; forcibly conscripted or recruited; subjected to torture, rape and mutilation; forced to commit sexual violence upon others	
	Higher rates of disability from injury	
Women	Higher likelihood to be internally displaced persons and refugees	Reproductive health problems
	Sexual and gender-based violence: being subjected to rape	Women's reproductive and care-giving roles under stress
	Trafficking and prostitution; forced pregnancies and marriages	Changed labour market participation from death of family members and 'added worker effect'
		Higher incidence of domestic violence
		Possibility for greater political participation
		Increased economic participation due to changing gender roles during conflict.

Common	Depression, trauma, and emotional distress	Asset and income loss
		Tendency toward increased migration
		Disrupted patterns of marriage and fertility
		Loss of family and social networks, including insurance mechanisms
		Interrupted education
		Eroded well-being, particularly poor health and disability from poverty and malnutrition.

Displaced populations

One of the most disruptive effects of conflict on society is population displacement. **Forced displacement** refers to people being forced to leave their homes due to violence, conflict, persecution, and human rights violations. **Displaced persons** leave behind homes, livelihoods and most possessions. Families may become separated while fleeing danger, or lose loved ones during fighting. They can be exhausted and disoriented from travelling long distances in search of refuge and suffering from malnutrition. Many will suffer psychosocial effects of trauma and social upheaval. Many may have lost important legal documents (e.g. identity cards, marriage licences, property ownership papers, birth certificates, school diplomas).

Displaced people are categorized as either **refugees** or **internally displaced persons (IDPs)** depending on whether they have crossed international borders or remain within their country of origin. At the end of 2009, the World Bank reported that 42 million people globally had been displaced due to conflict, violence, or human rights violations, while 10.2 million refugees sought refuge in developing countries, straining already scarce resources among host communities (World Bank, 2011).

The 1951 Refugee Convention defines a refugee as someone who 'owing to a well-founded fear of being persecuted for reasons of race, religion, nationality, membership of a particular social group or political opinion is outside the country of his nationality, and is unable to, or owing to such fear, is unwilling to avail himself of the protection of that country'. International refugee law provides for the protection and assistance of refugees from the international community and host countries to which refugees have moved.

According to the 1998 UN Guiding Principles on Internal Displacement, IDPs are 'persons or groups of persons who have been forced or obliged to flee or to leave their homes or places of habitual residence, in particular as a result of or in order to avoid the effects of armed conflict, situations of generalized violence, violations of human rights or natural or human-made disaster, and who have not crossed an internationally recognized State border'. Although IDPs remain entitled to all the rights and guarantees of citizens of their home country, it is often precisely due to a lack of human rights that they were forced to flee.

An influx of displaced persons places a burden on the **host community**. Community members may see refugees and IDPs as a drain on already meagre community resources. Additionally, external assistance provided to displaced populations can foster resentment among host communities, who may themselves be among the most marginalized segments of their own society.

Unlike refugees and IDPs, migrants choose to move in an attempt to improve their lives. Increasing numbers of economic migrants travel in search of better opportunities in more affluent parts of the globalized world. According to the International Organization for Migration (IOM), **mixed migration** refers to complex population movements (e.g. refugees, asylum seekers, economic and other migrants) in which migrants leave their home countries for a combination of reasons fundamentally related to safeguarding physical and economic security. Distinguishing between these groups is increasingly difficult as many individuals change status en route. For example, an IDP in one country may seek refugee status in a neighbouring country and then move to a third country as a migrant seeking employment and a better standard of life. As with displaced persons, these migrants may be vulnerable to human rights violations, including human trafficking.

While assessing vulnerable population groups, it is important to consider resilience and potentially resilient groups. Being elderly, female, or disabled, does not automatically make someone more vulnerable during conflict. For example, an elderly person who is able to get help and support from family and social networks during crises will be more resilient than someone with insufficient income and social support. Likewise, marginalized religious or ethnic groups may have developed effective coping strategies prior to conflict (e.g. cultural traditions, access to resources, social support) that foster community resilience.

Activity 2.2

The UN Convention on the Rights of the Child was adopted in 1959 to protect children caught in conflicts throughout the world. It states:

> The child shall enjoy special protection, and shall be given opportunities and facilities, by law and by other means, to enable him to develop physically, mentally, morally, spiritually and socially in a healthy and normal manner and in conditions of freedom and dignity. In the enactment of laws for this purpose, the interests of the child will be the paramount consideration.

2.2.1 Briefly describe why children are particularly vulnerable to the effects of conflict.

2.2.2 Identify the types of violations that are often committed against children during conflict.

Challenges to basic needs

Shelter

When people are forced from their homes they require transitional shelter, which should provide 'a habitable covered living space and a secure, healthy living environment, with privacy and dignity to those within it, during the period between a conflict or natural disaster and the achievement of a durable shelter solution' (Vitale and Corsellis, 2005). Displaced populations often take refuge in a **transitional settlement**.

Transitional settlements can be either grouped or dispersed. Displaced populations often choose grouped settlements for security, to support communal coping strategies, and to access aid and resources (Vitale and Corsellis, 2005). However, according to UN High Commissioner for Refugees (UNHCR) figures, only one-third of the world's 10.5 million refugees live in camps, while more than half migrate to urban areas.

Grouped transitional settlements occur when displaced people settle together. Three main types of grouped settlements are collective centres, self-settled camps, and planned camps. Collective centres, also called mass shelters, are often transit facilities located in large pre-existing structures (e.g. community centres, town halls, gymnasiums, hotels, warehouses, abandoned factories) (Vitale and Corsellis, 2005). Self-settled camps occur when displaced communities settle together, independent of assistance from local government or humanitarian agencies (Vitale and Corsellis, 2005). Planned camps, often organized by international humanitarian agencies in partnership with host governments, provide accommodation and dedicated infrastructure (e.g. food aid, sanitation, health facilities). Displaced populations, particularly IDPs, may be settled in isolated or undesirable areas, where resources such as clean water and fertile land are scarce, the potential for formal or informal employment restricted, they are exposed to landmines or explosive remnants of war, or face increased marginalization and hostility as targets for abuse and attack (Sphere, 2011). Conditions in organized settlements can be damaging to physical, psychological and social well-being. Camps are often overcrowded, leading to a lack of privacy and public health problems.

Dispersed transitional settlements occur when displaced persons settle informally within host communities. Three types of dispersed settlements are dispersal to host families (i.e. displaced individuals or families take shelter in the homes of local families), rural self-settlement (i.e. settlement on rural, collectively owned land), and urban self-settlement (i.e. settling informally in an urban environment, occupying unclaimed properties or land). In all circumstances, there is often heavy reliance on the host community, friends or family for assistance and support. Tracing dispersed populations can be challenging, while services and support are harder to provide than in a camp setting. However, dispersed settlement is considered more sustainable as it can offer displaced families opportunities to stay anonymous, earn money, and be less dependent on external support.

Awareness of different types of transitional settlements helps in delivering effective health programming for vulnerable displaced populations. For example, an **immunization campaign** targeting displaced children under 2 years of age will be delivered differently in a planned camp than in a dispersed settlement where children are cared for by host families.

Security

A primary concern among conflict-affected and displaced populations is some sense of security. IHL, also known as the **law of war**, aims to protect persons who are not or are no longer taking part in hostilities (e.g. the sick, the wounded, prisoners, civilians) and define the rights and obligations of conflicting parties in the conduct of hostilities. IHL governs relations between states in times of conflict, and relies on an evolving body of law including the Geneva and Hague Conventions. The **Responsibility to Protect** is an internationally recognized norm highlighting government responsibility to protect its citizens from grave human rights violations (e.g. genocide). In cases where a government is considered unable to protect its citizens or is perpetrating these crimes, the international community has the responsibility to intervene. Chapter 11 will discuss security and protection in more depth.

Activity 2.3

The following quote is taken from an Amnesty International report (Amnesty International, 2004): 'the majority of IDPs live in spontaneous camps and settlements around the cities or large villages of Darfur, where they continue to be the target of attacks, killings, rapes and harassment by the Janjawid, whose presence is reported in the cities or at the periphery of the IDP camps'. Explain how the situation described in the report constitutes a breakdown of the rule of law.

Food

Food security is defined in many ways, including the widely accepted 1996 World Food Summit definition 'when all people, at all times, have physical, social and economic access to sufficient, safe and nutritious food to meet their dietary needs and food preferences for an active and healthy life' (Sphere, 2011). Conflicts often occur in countries experiencing chronic food insecurity (Egal, 2006). Humanitarian interventions during conflict often respond quickly to food shortages with programming that may include general food distribution, supplementary feeding, micronutrient supplementation, and nutrition education associated with health services. Chapter 9 provides further discussion of nutrition in conflict-affected settings.

Water, sanitation, and hygiene (WASH)

Conflict can contribute to water scarcity in a community through contamination of water sources or destruction of infrastructure such as wells, reservoirs and pipes. Population displacement can also affect the water needs of a community. If large numbers of displaced persons arrive in a community that already suffers from water shortages, the increased consumption will place an added burden on the local water system and potentially increase hostility in the host community.

Populations with insufficient water quality and quantity will face severe health risks, additionally stressing health systems. Lack of sufficient drinking water quality will lead to increases in diarrhoeal disease morbidity and mortality. Lack of sufficient water quantities for sanitation (e.g. excreta disposal), hygiene (e.g. hand-washing), and agriculture can lead to increased morbidity and mortality from diarrhoeal diseases and malnutrition. Chapter 8 provides further discussion of diarrhoeal diseases.

Livelihoods

According to the **non-governmental organization** Oxfam, **livelihood** describes how people routinely earn money to meet basic family needs and its loss is one of the most devastating effects of conflict on families. Livelihoods are central to coping during non-emergency times, but are also a key part of coping during and recovering after crises. People who lose their livelihoods are less able to provide for basic needs for themselves and their families, thereby increasing their vulnerability.

Loss of livelihood can manifest in different economic and psychosocial ways. People who rely on subsistence farming as their means of livelihood may be forced to abandon land and crops, leaving them without food or shelter. Conflict encourages economic migration whereby people, often men, leave their families and relocate to find work. Loss of livelihood increases vulnerability to military recruitment, sex work, and theft. Women who have lost husbands or relatives during conflict may assume economic responsibility for their family in addition to fulfilling domestic duties. Supply chains of goods and services will be severely affected when businesses close and transport routes are disrupted. Professionals (e.g. doctors, teachers) may leave for other countries, reducing the educated workforce and population access to needed services.

Maintaining or re-establishing livelihoods is so crucial for conflict-affected populations that it has become a cornerstone of humanitarian programming. Humanitarian livelihood initiatives are varied, but aim to generate income for conflict-affected communities while supporting self-reliance and resilience. Examples of livelihood programmes include food-for-work projects that support road building and land clearance, micro-credit loans to entrepreneurs, seed and tool distribution, and incentive payments to health workers for immunization campaigns.

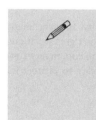

Activity 2.4

Although displaced populations are considered a vulnerable group, there are ways they can increase their own resilience to the negative effects of conflict.
2.4.1 Give two examples of humanitarian programmes that could increase resilience in displaced populations.
2.4.2 Briefly explain how these two programmes would affect vulnerability.

Conclusions

This chapter began with an overview of the effects of conflict on human development, examined concepts of vulnerability and resilience, and described ways conflict affects basic needs of society, including shelter, security, food, and water. The social, economic and political effects of conflict are complex and long lasting. Conflict can disrupt human development by limiting access to basic needs, particularly for marginalized groups. Two of the most disruptive effects of conflict on society are forced displacement and loss of livelihoods. The next chapter examines specific effects of conflict on health, including mortality and morbidity rates.

Feedback on activities

Feedback on Activity 2.1

2.1.1 You might have looked at economic data, such as GDP. You might also have considered that economic assessment cannot account for psychological, cultural, and environmental costs and looked at ways to assess these costs (e.g.

collecting and analysing health indicators, education and literacy rates, mental health statistics, HDI, and even primary community research).

2.1.2 HDI is a composite statistic combining life expectancy, literacy, education, and standards of living. It is used to rank countries according to level of well-being and development. Thus, a country with a low HDI ranking would be considered underdeveloped and might experience high levels of poverty and social inequality, poor educational achievement, and low life expectancy.

Feedback on Activity 2.2

2.2.1 You may have described how children are particularly physically and psychologically vulnerable to the effects of conflict due to physical and mental immaturity and their dependence on adults.

2.2.2 According to the UN Special Representative of the Secretary-General for Children and Armed Conflict, the six grave violations against children during conflict are: (i) killing or maiming of children, (ii) recruitment or use of child soldiers, (iii) rape and other forms of sexual violence against children, (iv) abduction of children, (v) attacks against schools or hospitals, and (vi) denial of humanitarian access to children (Kolieb and Tasheebeva, 2009). You may have identified some or all of these violations.

Feedback on Activity 2.3

You might have said that this represents a breakdown of the rule of law as government did not provide IDPs with law and order or protect them from human rights violations (Belton, 2009). Sexual violence was used to control and humiliate the community, suggesting that in this example the government failed in its responsibility to protect its citizens.

Feedback on Activity 2.4

2.4.1 You could have identified a number of programmes, including those for livelihood, peer education, and psychosocial support.

2.4.2 Depending on your selection, these two programmes could affect vulnerability by, for example, increasing household income, improving general education indicators, and strengthening household resilience.

Effects of conflict on health

Natasha Howard, Mazeda Hossain and Lara Ho

Overview

The aim of this chapter is to examine the health effects of conflict, focusing on excess mortality and morbidity and disease burden from direct and indirect effects. Concepts from the health security literature and epidemiological research in conflict-affected settings are used to examine the health effects of conflict.

Learning outcomes

When you have completed this chapter, you should be able to:

- describe the effects of conflict on mortality, morbidity, and disability outcomes
- consider risk factors and direct and indirect consequences of conflict
- calculate basic epidemiological measures to assess health outcomes in conflict-affected settings

Effects of conflict on health outcomes

Physical and psychological injuries, malnutrition, infectious disease outbreaks, and **excess mortality** are the devastating health outcomes experienced by combatants and non-combatants during and after periods of violent conflict. Factors that influence the immediate and lasting effects of conflict on health include the nature, intensity and duration of conflict violence, pre-existing development levels and health status, and commitment to reconstruction efforts.

Health outcomes of conflict can be categorized as increased mortality, morbidity and disability. Table 3.1 summarizes the effects of conflict violence on health outcomes, including potential causes and examples in each category.

Mortality

Mortality rates are often used as an **indicator** of the damage caused by violent conflict. Total conflict mortality combines battle deaths and indirect deaths from conflict-exacerbated malnutrition and disease. While numbers of wars, conflicts and genocides are relatively well documented, resulting deaths are difficult to count (Human Security Report Project, 2011). Unsurprisingly, measurement of deaths due to conflict is not straightforward and may be disputed, as different definitions are used for different purposes (Coghlan et al., 2009). Despite this, conflict-related mortality offers a way to measure the impact of conflict on a population and compare it with other conflicts.

Table 3.1 Effects of conflict violence on health outcomes

Health outcomes	Potential causes	Examples
Increased mortality	External physical trauma	• Weapons attack, physical and sexual violence
	Infectious diseases	• Malaria, tetanus, diarrhoeal diseases
	Preventable non-communicable diseases and emergencies avoided through health care access	• Asthma, diabetes, emergency surgery, maternal and neonatal mortality
Increased morbidity	Injuries due to physical trauma	• Weapons attack, burns, mutilation, sexual and physical violence
	Infectious diseases	• Water-related (cholera, typhoid, dysentery), sexually transmitted (HIV, other sexually transmitted infections), vaccine-preventable (tuberculosis, measles, mumps, meningococcal meningitis), vector-borne (malaria, viral haemorrhagic fevers), acute respiratory infections (pneumonia)
	Chronic and non-infectious diseases	• Lack of supportive treatment for long-term illnesses (e.g. cancers, hypertension, HIV)
	Reproductive and sexual disorders	• Increased stillbirths, prematurity/low birthweight, delivery complications, unintended/forced pregnancy, traumatic genital fistula
	Malnutrition	• Acute and chronic malnutrition, vitamin and nutrient deficiencies
	Mental distress	• Anxiety, depression, suicidal ideation
Increased disability	Reduced physical functioning	• Permanent injuries due to loss of limbs or mutilation, disability due to lack of vaccination programmes
	Mental disorders	• Acute and chronic psychoses, epilepsy, alcohol and substance misuse, severe emotional disorders, post-traumatic stress disorder, common mental disorders
	Reduced social engagement	• Isolation from resources, for those disabled prior to conflict, due to lack of accessible transport or loss of community support

Source: adapted from Krug et al. (2002), Medact (2004), Mont and Loeb (2008), Jones et al. (2009) and Connolly et al. (2004).

Collection and publication of crude and excess mortality rates can be useful alongside cause-specific mortality rates (e.g. diarrhoeal diseases, malnutrition) that provide a better picture of the impact of the conflict on health (Degomme and Guha-Sapir, 2010). The University of Uppsala has developed a database of reported deaths from conflict violence globally. These reported deaths must meet stringent criteria, so results are lower than actual deaths. However, Uppsala's counts allow calculation of yearly

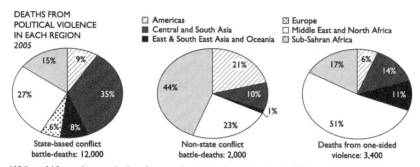

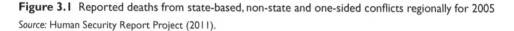

While useful for tracking trneds, these figrues underestimate the real death tolls. This is particularly true in the case of Iraq, where fatality estimates are wildly divergent and intensely controversial.

Figure 3.1 Reported deaths from state-based, non-state and one-sided conflicts regionally for 2005
Source: Human Security Report Project (2011).

trends, geographical spread, and relative lethality of the main forms of organized political violence (Human Security Report Project, 2011).

Morbidity

As with mortality rates, total morbidity combines direct battle injuries and indirect morbidities of disease, malnutrition, collateral injuries and mental trauma. Indirect morbidity is considerably higher than direct morbidity. For most settings, there is little publically available information on the extent of civilians and combatants who have been injured or fallen ill as a direct result of conflict violence (Medact, 2004). As **humanitarian assistance** has become increasingly professionalized and cost-effective since the end of the Cold War, a major focus has been on reducing morbidity and thus mortality from the four major disease threats – diarrhoeal diseases, acute respiratory infections, malaria and measles – that can be prevented and treated at low cost (Human Security Report Project, 2011).

Disability

Conflict-related disability has sometimes been included with morbidity statistics and fewer data are available about the effects of conflict on disability in comparison to data on mortality outcomes. A key difference that distinguishes disability from morbidity is the focus on physical and mental functioning. We can define disability as a physical or mental condition that limits a person's movements, senses, or activities, often permanently or over long periods of time. Disabilities may precede conflict and potentially contribute to vulnerability, or may be caused or exacerbated by conflict (e.g. loss of limbs, post-traumatic stress disorder) and can cause substantial functional impairment (Kett and van Ommeren, 2009; Mont and Loeb, 2008). During and immediately after conflict, limited resources will likely be focused on the most pressing morbidities, which may not include long-term trauma related to experiences of conflict or related violence.

Activity 3.1

Choose two ongoing conflicts in which you are interested. Consider how you would compare the health impact of the two conflicts, using freely available online data. What kinds of information would you try to collect?

Health risk factors and consequences of conflict

Risk factors

Health risk factors may be categorized as proximate, intermediate or distal. The relationship of conflict morbidity and mortality to immediate proximate risk factors, such as exposure to unsafe water or disease vectors, is often obvious. However, it can be more challenging to trace these back to distal factors such as economic stagnation or environmental vulnerability. Figure 3.2 provides a cognitive framework for commonly considered risk factors.

Direct and indirect health consequences

Direct consequences of conflict include battle deaths and injuries. Indirect consequences are much broader and more difficult to estimate. Much conflict-related research has been focused on mortality, which may be partially attributable to the

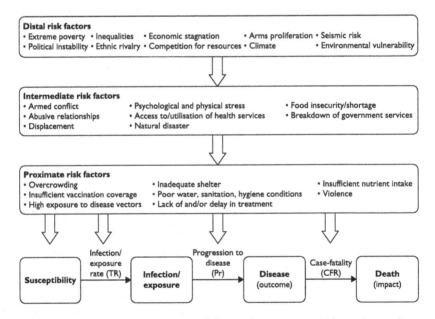

Figure 3.2 Distal, intermediate and proximate risk factors for excess morbidity and mortality in a conflict
Source: Checchi et al. (2007).

complexities of understanding cumulative and often complicated interactions between an individual's experience and their setting (Spiegel et al., 2010b). Clarifying causal pathways between the destruction of a country's infrastructure, individual experiences of violence, levels of violence in the community and gender-specific issues is not straightforward. Despite these difficulties, various violence and associated health-related assessments have been completed among survivors, who are often victims of severe and multiple forms of physical, sexual and psychological violence (Watts et al., 2010).

In 2012, conflicts of varying size continued in countries as varied as the Democratic Republic of Congo (DRC), Angola, Iraq, Yemen, Afghanistan, and Myanmar (Uppsala Universitet, 2012). For example, one analysis of mortality indicators in Darfur found that although deaths attributable to violence increased in 2004 due to displacement and attacks, the decrease in subsequent years remained in excess of the expected mortality rate. This excess mortality noted in 2006–7 is most likely attributable to indirect causes such as preventable or treatable diseases and the declining provision of services by humanitarian organizations (Checchi, 2010; Degomme and Guha-Sapir, 2010).

Indirect health consequences can be positive or negative, depending on the nature of the conflict and setting. For example, a violent war may lead to a decrease in mortality in the long term when war-related violence, such as mass killings, is finally halted (Murray et al., 2002), the displacement of a population can lead to a decrease in levels of HIV or other sexually transmitted infections rather than an increase (Watts et al., 2010), or levels of intimate partner violence or community violence can increase in the post-conflict period.

Health system consequences

As with other forms of collective violence, conflict causes injuries among participating combatants and those caught up in the combat. Both threatened and actual conflict violence can affect the health system and health care delivery in several ways. First, health care facilities and staff may be attacked directly or bombed accidentally. Second, active fighting near health centres can prevent access by staff and patients needing care. It can block service vehicles and ambulances and disrupt electrical and water services. Third, conflict violence can forcibly displace non-combatants, including health care personnel, to safer areas. Fourth, conflict and violence can hamper implementation of preventive services, such as vaccination campaigns.

Activity 3.2

How might you distinguish health risks and consequences of a protracted or chronic conflict from those in an acute conflict?

Epidemiological assessment of conflict

Health **assessment** in conflict-affected settings is differentiated from more stable settings primarily by the lack of national-level data, difficulties in collecting accurate and representative data, and breakdown of health and social services and infrastructure. Basic epidemiological indicators are useful in assessing health outcomes. They can describe mortality (e.g. mortality rates, excess mortality) and morbidity or disability (e.g. **incidence, prevalence**, losses in life expectancy or quality). To be understandable, indicators should always describe person, place and time (e.g. '14% of children aged 0–5 years in Dadaab refugee camp in 2013'). The three main types of indicators used are proportions, ratios and rates.

Proportions are calculated as A/N, where A is part of N, and are often presented as percentages. For example, if you are told that among 100 infants in a refugee camp, 32 were found to be stunted during a recent nutrition survey, you can calculate the prevalence of stunting among these infants as $32/100 = 0.32$ or 32%. Thus, 32% of infants in this refugee camp were found to be stunted during the survey.

Ratios are calculated as A/B, where A is not part of B. For example, if you are told that 20% of IDPs and 10% of the host population in your area have been diagnosed with malaria during a weekly survey, you can calculate the prevalence ratio as $0.20/0.10 = 2.0$. Thus, IDPs in your area were twice as likely to be diagnosed with malaria as were members of the host population during that week.

Rates are calculated as $A/N \times$ Person $\times$ Time-period. For example, if you are told that 7 patients died out of 350 patients seen at the health centre yesterday, you can calculate the mortality rate as $7/350 = 0.02$ or 2 per 100 per day. Multiplied by 10,000, this means the **crude mortality rate** is 200 per 10,000 people per day and thus over the consensual threshold used to indicate an emergency.

Table 3.2 provides common mortality indicators used to estimate health outcomes and impact from conflict. Of these, the most widely reported is probably excess mortality. Excess mortality calculations quantify deaths due to the conflict, thus providing an objective indication of severity and health impact. The crude mortality rate is often used to demonstrate the scale and intensity of a conflict and is the key public health indicator used in crisis monitoring, though it is not adjusted for age or sex.

Table 3.2 Common mortality indicators used in conflict settings

Indicator	Basic formula	Applications and interpretation
Crude mortality rate (CMR)	Number of deaths from all causes/ (Population at risk × Time-period)	Usually expressed as deaths per 10,000 people per day; CMR > 1/10,000 per day indicates an emergency
Group-specific mortality rate	Number of deaths by age or population group/(Population at risk × Time-period)	Usually calculated for particularly vulnerable groups (e.g. children under age 5, IDPs). Similar calculations can be used for period-specific and disease-specific mortality rates
Proportional mortality	Number of cause-specific deaths/ Total number of deaths	Usually expressed as a percentage in community or health facilities; helps determine health priorities
Case fatality rate	Number of cause-specific deaths/ Total number of cause-specific cases	Used to determine the probability of dying from a particular disease or cause (i.e. lethality)
Excess mortality rate	Observed mortality rate – Expected non-crisis mortality rate (× At-risk population × Time-period)	Used as an objective indicator of crisis severity

Source: Adapted from information supplied by F. Checchi.

Table 3.3 Morbidity and disability indicators used in conflict settings

Individual/group level	Basic formula	Applications and interpretation
Incidence rate	Number of new cases/Total population × Time-period	Used to determine whether morbidity is increasing
Prevalence	Number of cases/Total population at a point or short period in time	Used as an estimate of how common an outcome is in a population and time-point of interest
Proportional morbidity	Number of cause-specific clinic visits/Total number of clinic visits	Usually expressed as a percentage in community or health facilities; helps determine health priorities
Excess morbidity rate	Observed morbidity rate – Expected non-crisis morbidity rate × (At-risk population × Time-period)	Used as an objective indicator of crisis severity
Population level		
Years of life lost (YLL)	Number of deaths × Standard life expectancy at age of death in years	A traditional measure of disease burden that does not account for disability
Years lost to disability (YLD)	Number of incident cases × Disability weight × Average years duration until remission or death	A measurement of disability burden
Disability-adjusted life years (DALYs)	YLL + YLD	A simple, popular metric used to assess impact on disability and premature mortality
Quality-adjusted life-years (QALYs)	Year of life × Utility value	A measurement of disease burden combining quantity and perceived quality of life
Healthy life years (HLYs)	Life expectancy – Expected number of years lived with chronic activity limitations	A more recent structural indicator, intended to capture both mortality and ill-health

Source: Adapted from information supplied by F. Checchi.

Table 3.3 provides common indicators used to estimate morbidity and disability outcomes and impact from conflict. Individual and group-level indicators are also useful in programme monitoring, while population-level indicators are more difficult to calculate, rely on consensual but arbitrary decisions on disability weights, and are used most commonly for international advocacy, resource allocation and aid rationalization.

Activity 3.3

You are working as a health advisor in an acute emergency. Your field team found an 'excess mortality' of 0.7/10,000 per day in No. 8 Refugee Camp and you have requested additional supplies. However, your regional manager insists that the

NGO can only provide extra supplies if the crude mortality rate surpasses the emergency threshold of 1/10,000 per day and baseline crude mortality for this population is assumed to be 0.5/10,000 per day.

3.3.1 What would you advise the field team to do?
3.3.2 How would you justify this to your regional manager?

Conclusions

This chapter began with an overview of the effects of conflict on health outcomes, described examples of direct and indirect consequences of conflict on health systems, and considered health outcome assessment in conflict-affected settings. The next chapter will examine international responses to conflict.

Feedback on activities

Feedback on Activity 3.1

You may have found a number of good data sources. Two sources at the time of writing are the Uppsala University Conflict Database (UCDB) and the Human Security Report Project (HSRP) and its *miniAtlas of Human Security*. The UCDB (http://www.ucdp.uu.se/gpdatabase/search.php) maps an annual breakdown of war, non-state, and one-sided conflicts. The HSRP (http://www.hsrgroup.org/) tracks global and regional trends in organized violence, including causes and consequences.

Feedback on Activity 3.2

You might have said that in a protracted conflict, in addition to high direct and indirect mortality, lack of governance, health system collapse and infrastructural breakdown lead to increasingly poor health outcomes and life expectancy.

Feedback on activity 3.3

3.3.1 You would probably advise them to provide the needed supplies to No. 8 Refugee Camp.
3.3.2 You could explain that excess mortality is defined as that part of mortality caused by the crisis additional to assumed normal mortality, thus there appears to have been confusion about the difference between crude and excess mortality. The baseline mortality rate should be added to the excess mortality rate. Therefore, we have a crude mortality rate of 0.5 + 0.7 = 1.2 per 10,000 per day, which is over the emergency threshold. The **emergency threshold** is actually defined as a doubling of normal (non-conflict) mortality for that region. The consensual threshold of 1/10,000 per day to indicate crisis is actually based on a doubling of the normal mortality rate found in many low-income countries.

International responses to conflict

Valerie Percival

Overview

The aim of this chapter is to provide an overview of international responses to conflict, focusing on key actors and approaches. Concepts from the international relations literature and policy analysis in conflict-affected settings are used to examine international responses to conflict.

Learning outcomes

After completing this chapter you should be able to:

* identify the rationales, key approaches and main actors that shape international engagement in conflict settings
* describe how health interventions in conflict fit within the broader international response
* analyse the key debates regarding health action in conflict-affected settings

International engagement in conflict settings

The rationale for engagement

The number of conflicts worldwide is declining, the number of war deaths has fallen, and civilian casualties appear to be decreasing (Goldstein, 2011; Human Security Report Project, 2011). One explanation for this decline is the active engagement of the international community in conflict-affected states, particularly the use of preventive diplomacy, humanitarian assistance to civilians, and peace-keeping missions (Human Security Report Project, 2011). Many analysts credit the deployment of integrated peace-keeping or stabilization missions, in which the UN and other multilateral agencies deploy peace-keeping and political resources simultaneously, for reducing both the impact of conflict on civilians and the overall rate of violent conflict (Human Security Report Project, 2011). However, while the aggregate numbers of civilians killed, injured, or otherwise affected by violence may be declining, for civilians living within conflict-affected regions it remains a key determinant of increased morbidity and mortality.

The active engagement of the international community in conflict-affected countries (i.e. states in political discourse) has increased since the end of the Cold War. The international community engages in these states for several reasons. First, states intervene to protect their own political or economic interests that could be threatened by an escalation of violence or the spread of conflict to neighbouring countries. As globalization heightens political and economic ties among countries, violence can have profound repercussions around the world. Second, membership in the UN, in military alliances such as the North Atlantic Treaty Organization (NATO), or other international organizations such as the Organization for Security and Cooperation in Europe (OSCE), the African Union (AU) or the European Union (EU) may oblige states to support various forms of international engagement. Third, while evidence shows that many states emerging from war are prone to **recidivism** – the return to violent conflict – the active engagement of the international community in some states has reduced the risks of further instability. As a result, some members of the international community have recognized the value of early and active involvement in states affected by violence and emerging from war. Finally, states and groups of states may engage in conflict-affected states in response to an escalation of human rights abuses and the deliberate targeting of civilians. In such states, the international community may evoke the evolving norm of *responsibility to protect*. This norm, mentioned in Chapter 2, was first formally raised by the International Commission on Intervention and State Sovereignty, formed in the wake of the Kosovo war, and subsequently integrated into the UN General Assembly's World Summit Outcome Document of 2005. It has been referenced in several UN Security Council Resolutions (UNSCRs), including UNSCR 1769 that established the AU–UN hybrid mission in Darfur; UNSCR 1856 that expanded the mandate of the UN peace-keeping mission in the Democratic Republic of Congo (DRC); and UNSCR 1973 that established the no-fly zone in Libya. According to this norm, when the state is unable to protect its civilians from grave abuses of human rights, or when the state is the actor committing those abuses, the international community has an obligation to intervene diplomatically and militarily.

Stages and tools of international engagement

There are generally three stages of international engagement in conflict-affected states – prevention, containment and active intervention. First, to *prevent* violence from escalating, the international community attempts to persuade conflicting parties to abide by international law, undertake political reforms and commit to processes to resolve their differences. Second, once conflict has escalated, the international community may work to *mitigate or contain* the impact of conflict. Third, if the first two have failed, the international community can undertake *active intervention* to resolve the conflict.

To prevent, mitigate and resolve conflict, the international community uses four basic tools. These are diplomacy, humanitarian assistance, military intervention, and development assistance (e.g. reconstruction and **early recovery** assistance).

Diplomacy, the art of persuasion, is often used to prevent the escalation of conflict. Diplomatic envoys attempt to convince states and **non-state actors** to undertake particular political, social and economic measures within the state, or to participate in political, social and economic activities in the international arena. These diplomatic messages can be conveyed by representatives from states, through coordinated diplomatic pressure from like-minded states, and also through representatives of international organizations. In the context of conflict-affected states, diplomacy includes fact-finding missions and observer groups; resolutions of the United Nations Security Council and General Assembly reminding conflicting parties of their obligations under international humanitarian law; special envoys who mediate among conflicting parties and outline the parameters of a potential resolution to the conflict; and communication of the consequences if a state does not change its behaviour. Such warnings fall under the rubric of coercive diplomacy, and include the issuing of credible threats of economic sanctions, freezing of assets, expulsion from regional or multilateral organizations, and the threat of force.

Humanitarian assistance is the provision of life-saving assistance to civilians, whose health and well-being are threatened when conflict, violence or natural disasters have disrupted the supply of food, shelter, health care, and access to water and sanitation. **Humanitarian actors** engage in the direct delivery of emergency life-saving services, including provision of food, water, medical assistance and shelter. Funding time-frames are measured in weeks and months, with humanitarian action focused on the rapid alleviation of morbidity and mortality.

Military intervention is the active deployment of military forces, often supplemented by other representatives of the security sectors such as the police, to monitor and enforce the terms of a peace agreement (e.g. Bosnia, Kosovo), protect civilians from the actions of warring parties (e.g. Darfur, DRC), or actively take sides in a conflict (e.g. Afghanistan, Libya). While military intervention can occasionally be unilateral, most often it is undertaken by coalitions of like-minded states, often led by one dominant country (e.g. the United States in Iraq), by regional organizations such as NATO (e.g. Bosnia, Kosovo, Afghanistan, Libya), through regional organizations (e.g. the Economic Community of West African States in Sierra Leone, the EU in Chad), or multilateral organizations (e.g. the UN peace-keeping missions). If the UN Security Council determines that such action falls under the mandate of Chapter VII of the UN Charter, and is necessary for 'international peace and security', the Security Council can author-ize UN peace-keeping missions to use force (e.g. DRC, Darfur).

Development assistance is a form of active international intervention in conflict-affected states. Funding is often provided for one or more years. Given the destruction of infrastructure that accompanies conflict, donors provide often significant resources for the repair and rebuilding of critical infrastructure, including roads, water distribu-tion and purification, sanitation systems, schools, and health facilities. To reverse some of the causes of state fragility and reduce the risk of recidivism, the international com-munity has recognized the need to go beyond the provision of reconstruction aid. These activities, labelled *early recovery*, include initial efforts to build and strengthen the institutions of government, to reform and establish civilian oversight of the security sector (including the military and the police), to build political parties that can engage in democratic processes, and to strengthen civic participation. The objective is to establish sustainable, nationally owned initiatives that are focused on restoring basic services, securing livelihoods, advancing security and the rule of law, building governance mechanisms, and strengthening civil society.

Institutional actors in conflict

The global public policy agenda is crowded, with many issues vying for attention. How is a conflict-affected state elevated onto the global public policy agenda? Key actors involved in this process include states with an active diplomatic presence that are committing financial resources to humanitarian, development and military activities; the UN; other multilateral agencies involved in political and humanitarian efforts; advocacy groups; **international NGOs** providing humanitarian and development assistance; the military and private security firms; the conflict-affected state and conflict protagonists; and stakeholders within that state, including local NGOs. These actors and their role in the international response to conflict-affected states are summarized below.

National governments. Governments often have varying reasons for engaging in conflict-affected states, and the nature of their intervention varies accordingly. Often only a few states drive international engagement, allocate military resources, and provide funding for humanitarian and development assistance. For example, given their work with fragile and conflict-affected states, members of the UN Security Council are often actively engaged in policy development and set the international agenda for these states. Governments with commercial and economic interests at stake are also likely to engage in policy development. Some states, such as Norway, with a foreign policy that includes a commitment to human rights and human security, may choose to engage even in those states where the conflict has little impact on their national interest.

The United Nations. The UN, particularly the Security Council, is a key forum for putting conflict-affected states on the global public policy agenda and providing a mechanism for collective decision-making. At the Security Council, the five permanent members with veto power (the United States, Russia, China, France and the United Kingdom) and ten non-permanent members can request the UN Secretary-General to launch investigations into international disputes; issue recommendations on the settlement of these disputes; debate and determine threats to international peace and security and recommend particular action to address these threats; call on UN members to apply economic sanctions or other actions to address aggression; and authorize the use of force against aggressors. In addition, the UN Secretary-General is mandated to produce regular reports to the Security Council on progress made by UN peace-keeping missions.

If one or more permanent member of the Security Council vetoes a binding resolution advocating action in a conflict-affected state, the UN system offers other options. The UN Secretary-General can attempt to use his or her powers of diplomatic persuasion either personally or by appointing a special envoy for the conflict; the UN General Assembly can draft and vote on a non-binding resolution; and UN agencies can also take action, including resolutions and investigative reports by the UN Human Rights Council.

Multilateral organizations. UN specialized agencies are important actors in the humanitarian and developmental response. The Office for the Coordination of Humanitarian Affairs (OCHA), the World Health Organization (WHO), the UN High Commissioner for Refugees (UNHCR), UN Children's Fund (UNICEF), and UN Women are among the key actors engaged in policy development and programming in conflict-affected states. These agencies identify key priorities, provide technical assistance, define programmatic priorities, facilitate coordination among both international and local organizations, and raise funds from donor governments to implement programmes. The Inter-Agency Standing Committee on Emergencies (IASC), chaired by the head of OCHA, is a key actor – determining priorities and galvanizing action. The IASC is unique in that it also includes representatives from consortia of humanitarian NGOs as 'standing invitees'.

Advocacy groups and the media. International think tanks and the media can also put conflict-affected states on the international agenda. Through reporting and analysis, they shape how the conflict is framed, providing analyses and situation assessments to broader public audiences. Information technology makes the job of analysis and advocacy quicker and somewhat easier. When constrained by their inability to access certain conflict-affected states, technology such as crowd-source data enables the monitoring of crises from afar. For example, crisis mapping uses a combination of satellite images and crowd source data to provide critical details on population movements, troop movements, and the existence of mass graves.

Non-governmental organizations. Particularly in those states with disrupted infrastructure, NGOs deliver much-needed humanitarian, reconstruction, and early recovery assistance, sometimes in dangerous conditions. They can act as advocates, highlighting effects of the conflict on civilian populations, and raising funds for their operations directly from the public. While transnational/international NGOs have the highest profile, they rely on national NGOs to access civilians in insecure locations and understand local context and culture.

The military. Military actors, ranging from UN peace-keeping troops to soldiers posted to national and foreign conflicts, play various roles. First, they can act to monitor ceasefires of peace agreements, ensuring that warring parties do not violate the terms of their agreements. Second, they can participate in hostilities to enforce the terms of UNSCRs or the mandate outlined by organizations such as NATO. Third, they can take an active role in institution building, assisting in reform of the security sectors of conflict-affected states.

Private security firms. These actors have become common in conflict-affected states, particularly those with insurgent attacks against the international community. They are often used to protect diplomatic representatives and guard diplomatic offices, residences, and international NGO compounds. Individuals working for private security firms (PSFs) are often former members of the military, yet under international law they are not formally known as combatants and their status under international law remains unclear.

Conflict-affected states. The conflict-affected state is key to the international response, facilitating or impeding engagement with conflict protagonists or access to conflict-affected populations. Representatives of the conflict-affected state can also argue for international action through their positions at the UN General Assembly or regional organizations.

The role of health in international responses to conflict

Given the relationship between conflict and civilian morbidity and mortality, interventions to improve the health of populations are an important component of broader international engagement in conflict-affected states. Health engagement in conflict-affected states is a significant portion of both humanitarian aid and the reconstruction and early recovery components of development assistance.

Humanitarian assistance

Humanitarian assistance is the provision of life-saving interventions to civilian populations during war or natural disasters. Through years of delivering humanitarian aid, the international community has developed norms and coordination mechanisms to govern its delivery. These will be discussed in Chapter 5.

Health in humanitarian and early recovery responses

The health component of humanitarian assistance is significant, reported at approximately 9% of total assistance – in comparison, food aid is the largest component at 36.6% (Global Humanitarian Assistance, 2010). The two broad categories of health and medical assistance during humanitarian engagement are (i) mass immunization campaigns and (ii) provision of emergency health care services, delivered directly by international organizations or national NGOs. The growing evidence base in conflict settings has enhanced the effectiveness of international engagement in both assistance categories.

Immunization campaigns. Conflict and natural disasters can exacerbate the spread of infectious diseases through overcrowded conditions in refugee and internally displaced person camps, food insecurity and malnutrition, and the disruption of national health systems and WHO Expanded Programme on Immunization services. In some humanitarian contexts, infectious diseases such as measles are among the top causes of mortality, particularly among children. As many conflict-exacerbated diseases are preventable, mass vaccination campaigns are recommended as a priority intervention when population immunity is below the level needed to achieve **herd immunity**. Measles, for example, requires over 90% of the population to be immune to achieve this level. Immunization campaigns have been generally successful – for example, there was a 78% reduction in measles mortality from 2000 to 2008 (Grais et al., 2011). Immunization campaigns sometimes require health NGOs to negotiate ceasefires among protagonists to achieve sufficient population coverage. The most common immunizations used in humanitarian crises are measles, polio, BCG for tuberculosis, and DTP for diphtheria, tetanus and pertussis, while efforts are being made to include *Haemophilus influenzae* type b and hepatitis B vaccines.

Emergency health services. Humanitarian agencies deliver emergency health services consisting of **triage**, diagnosis and appropriate treatment. To ensure a professional, evidence-based response, the humanitarian community continues to develop and update technical guidelines through various forums on key elements of the medical response (e.g. the Sphere Standards, IASC guidelines).

Early recovery. In broader stabilization missions, the international community engages in the reconstruction and rebuilding of national **health systems**. WHO defines a health system as all the organizations, institutions, resources and people whose primary purpose is to improve health. Donors, in partnership with multilateral agencies and NGOs, rebuild health clinics and hospitals; propose the reorganization of health service delivery, emphasizing primary care; build financing systems to help achieve universal access to primary care services; train and supply health workers; and strengthen the capacity of governance oversight of health care delivery.

Rebuilding health systems is complex, particularly in humanitarian contexts characterized by weak governance, multiple public and private, international and national health-sector actors, and physical dangers. How can the donor community rebuild the capacity of the state, while simultaneously ensuring delivery of health care services? What health clinics should be rebuilt, and what services should they provide? How can the state sustainably finance universal access to primary health care services? How should the reform effort address the private health care sector, given the weak capacity of the state to regulate such services? The answers to these questions have been complicated by the dearth of research into health systems within the post-conflict environment.

Activity 4.1

You are an officer for a NATO contributing country, stationed in Kandahar, Afghanistan. Kandahar is at the heart of the Taliban insurgency in Afghanistan. The local hospital requires significant renovation to ensure the provision of running water and electricity to key sections of the hospital, including surgery and maternity units. You have the engineering staff and material resources to quickly undertake these repairs and are willing to offer these services pro bono. The WHO coordinator for the Kandahar region thanks you for your interest, but warns that any NATO engagement at the hospital will make it a target for insurgent attacks, placing staff and patients at risk. Senior NATO colleagues in Kabul agree that personnel must keep their distance from provision of emergency health services given humanitarian norms. However, they think the reconstruction of health facilities is not strictly humanitarian in nature and argue that it will win the 'hearts and minds' of local populations, thus helping quell support for the insurgency. When preparing your answers, consider the humanitarian principles of independence, impartiality and neutrality. You may wish to consult the IASC *Civil-Military Guidelines & Reference for Complex Emergencies* (IASC, 2008).

4.1.1 Do you think the reconstruction of a hospital, in the context of continuing violence and high levels of conflict, a humanitarian or development activity?
4.1.2 Do you think that humanitarian principles should apply to reconstruction projects?
4.1.3 What should be the parameters for military humanitarian operations in the context of peace-keeping or stabilization missions?

Debating health action in conflict

While the need to deliver life-saving assistance to civilians in need during humanitarian crises is not controversial, elements of the humanitarian response have generated significant debate. Key contentious issues are highlighted below.

Does humanitarian aid fuel conflict?

While the potential for humanitarian assistance to exacerbate conflict has been a constant concern, the response to the Rwandan genocide brought these issues to international attention. As the Rwandan Patriotic Front gradually halted the systematic slaughter of Tutsis through its invasion from Uganda in 1994, tens of thousands of Hutus fled to Zaire (now DRC). Accompanying civilians were members of the Interahamwe, the militia groups that led the planned and targeted killings of Tutsis. Using refugee camps in Zaire as their home base, they were fed and sheltered by the humanitarian community for several years until the Rwandan army invaded Zaire in 1997 (Terry, 2002). Humanitarian assistance undoubtedly helped the Interahamwe by providing food, shelter, protection as refugees, and the shelter of camps where they could find, indoctrinate and train new recruits. However, the issue is extremely complex for humanitarian actors.

Can the humanitarian community be held accountable for the resurgence of the Interahamwe? In the absence of that humanitarian assistance would the Interahamwe have disappeared as a fighting force? Moreover, what would have happened to the civilians – those non-combatants – who lived in the camps with the Interahamwe? Is it the job of the humanitarian community to separate combatants from non-combatants? What are the responsibilities of the humanitarian community when the international community will not act against combatants? While humanitarian assistance may play a role in exacerbating conflict, is the withdrawal of this assistance a choice that humanitarian actors can make, and how does it relate to the principle of **humanity** – the humane treatment of civilians in all circumstances through saving lives and alleviating suffering?

Humanitarian placebo

This debate is a variation on the issue of humanitarian assistance fuelling conflict. The international community often provides humanitarian aid to contain or mitigate the impact of conflict on civilian populations, in lieu of undertaking more forceful action to stop or reduce that impact. This is known as the **humanitarian placebo** – when humanitarian assistance is provided to civilian populations instead of a broader analysis of the causes and dynamics of the conflict and a political strategy that addresses those causes. Without this broader strategy, humanitarian assistance can inadvertently fuel conflict, as outlined above.

What does this mean for humanitarian actors? Should humanitarian actors resist efforts to provide humanitarian assistance to civilians in the absence of a broader political strategy to address the causes of violence? How would such a choice reflect on the principle of humanity?

Politicization of humanitarian assistance

The debate regarding the politicization of humanitarian assistance is closely related to the placebo debate, but at the opposite end of the spectrum. Whereas 'placebo' humanitarian aid is used *instead* of robust political action and a coherent strategy to address the root causes of violence, the politicization debate examines how the existence of a political strategy that guides international engagement in conflict-affected states *integrates* humanitarian assistance as a tool to achieve these broader political objectives. Key donor states fund humanitarian assistance to contribute to stability and/or to further their own economic or political objectives in conflict-affected states.

The politicization of humanitarian assistance occurs when **humanitarian principles of impartiality, neutrality** and **independence** are subordinated to political objectives. According to the Humanitarian Response Index, politicization manifests itself in various ways. Donor governments may link their support for humanitarian assistance to specific political or military objectives; prioritize long-term state-building goals over immediate humanitarian priorities; support the agendas set by recipient governments even when those governments have contributed to humanitarian crises; and use assistance to generate goodwill and support for either the international community or the recipient state.

To what extent is health assistance provided for political ends, and how does this impact on humanitarian actors and the recipients of humanitarian assistance? What is the middle ground between humanitarian assistance as a placebo, and the politicization of aid?

Use of international military personnel to deliver aid

Use of military actors to deliver humanitarian assistance is less problematic in natural disasters. However, in the context of fragile and conflict-affected states, military involvement in humanitarian assistance is highly contentious. While humanitarian actors are accustomed to navigating contexts with an active military presence, within the context of international engagement, where the international community has specific political objectives and uses military forces to achieve those objectives, the role of the military in humanitarian operations becomes complicated.

The military plays three main roles in humanitarian assistance. First, soldiers can work to provide a secure environment for humanitarian actors to provide assistance, while keeping a distance from humanitarian operations. Second, soldiers can actively protect humanitarian operations, guarding assistance conveys and ensuring the security and safety of specific locations where humanitarian assistance is provided. Third, soldiers can deliver humanitarian aid, either through direct assistance in the delivery of aid, or by providing medical care. Donor countries can also fund their militaries to provide humanitarian assistance.

Particularly in the context of stabilization and peace-keeping operations, the reason for the military to engage with local populations is clear – the delivery of assistance to civilian populations can build relationships with local communities and strengthen public support for the military presence. However, when military actors actively engage in the delivery of humanitarian aid – either by providing that assistance themselves or by closely associating themselves with that assistance – assistance is not being provided according to the humanitarian principles of independence, neutrality and impartiality.

Does the engagement of the military erode these principles for all humanitarian actors, as some humanitarian organizations argue?

The role of private security firms

The number of PSFs has risen dramatically in conflict-affected states, and most humanitarian organizations have employed them at some point. PSFs can be locally based or international, and can operate armed or unarmed. Most humanitarian organizations hire unarmed local PSFs, primarily to guard humanitarian offices, staff residences, aid storage facilities, and the delivery of humanitarian assistance. However, PSFs may have close contact with the military and police, eroding perceptions of the neutrality and independence of humanitarian organizations.

What is the appropriate legal status for these actors under international law? What are appropriate international norms for PSF best practices (Stoddard et al., 2009a)?

Corruption

During the humanitarian response, monitoring and accounting for the vast flows of material and financial assistance is extremely challenging. The context of humanitarian action – with its need for immediate life-saving assistance to be delivered in environments characterized by a breakdown of the rule of law, weak state capacity heightening the potential for abuse of authority, and powerful armed non-state actors who control access to land and people – does not facilitate accurate monitoring. In this context, humanitarian aid can be diverted and stolen, while significant bribes are sometimes paid to customs officials to secure the entry of assistance into the country and to local warlords to secure access to civilian populations.

Corruption has been a constant feature of humanitarian assistance, largely accepted as a cost of engaging in complex environments. However, its damaging consequences were highlighted by several recent events, which prompted the humanitarian community to reassess its response. The humanitarian response to the Rwandan genocide, the Iraq 'oil-for-food' programme that may have paid over US$1 billion in bribes from 1997 to 2003, and the corruption and pilfering of aid from recipient governments following the Indian Ocean tsunami brought the real costs of corruption to the fore (Maxwell et al., 2012). However, revelations of the human impact of corrupt and illegal practices have been far more disturbing than the financial costs of corruption. Reports documenting the sexual exploitation of children and women by peacekeeping troops and humanitarian officials in Guinea, Liberia and Sierra Leone showed how humanitarian actors can exploit their powerful positions in these contexts to abuse the most vulnerable in the humanitarian response (Maxwell et al., 2012).

There are a number of key questions defining this debate. What is the line between 'acceptable' levels of diversion of financial and material resources (e.g. corruption that is unavoidable given the context of humanitarian assistance) and unacceptable levels? When does corruption threaten the delivery of humanitarian assistance, diverting needed resources, and when does it facilitate that flow of resources to those in greatest need? What are the most effective mechanisms for humanitarian agencies to counter financial and material fraud collectively? How can the abuse of power by humanitarian officials be addressed effectively, given the weak state of the rule of law in countries experiencing humanitarian crises, and the limitations of national jurisdictions regarding the ability to prosecute their citizens for crimes committed abroad?

The role of national NGOs

International NGOs receive the most funding for humanitarian assistance, and are engaged in global decision-making processes regarding humanitarian assistance. However, national NGOs are critically important participants in the delivery of humanitarian assistance. They provide international NGOs with information on local contexts and culture; are implementing partners for the delivery of assistance, particularly when security conditions preclude the involvement of international actors; and can be funded to deliver that assistance, either by multilateral agencies or national donors, independent of the involvement of international NGOs. Although national NGOs are critical to the humanitarian response, there are several concerns. First, national NGOs represent a broad spectrum from well-established professional organizations, and very large and varied national Red Cross and Red Crescent membership societies, to small inexperienced or low-capacity organizations. Second, agendas can vary, from secular to faith-based, and ties to national and local governments or key conflict protagonists can be unclear. Third, during periods of high insecurity, when national NGOs are the only organizations capable of accessing affected populations, the ability of multilateral donor and partner organizations to monitor their activities is limited.

Given these conditions, how can the humanitarian community be certain that all national NGOs are abiding by **humanitarian norms**, and delivering assistance in an impartial manner?

Reconstruction and early recovery

The sustainability of humanitarian assistance has always been contentious. The humanitarian community is focused on immediate life-saving interventions that rapidly reduce civilian morbidity and mortality. Many humanitarian actors have avoided engaging in questions of sustainability, partly because of their narrow focus on short-term health improvements, but also because of humanitarian principles. A focus on the reconstruction and recovery of health systems involves engaging with the state in a manner that may jeopardize neutrality and independence, particularly if the state is a protagonist in the conflict. Moreover, state capacity is weak and reconstruction projects require significant sums of money. Safeguards against corruption must be built into these projects. Effective mechanisms and best practices for quickly improving health in a humanitarian context, while simultaneously strengthening health systems, have not yet been developed.

What are the long-term consequences of these humanitarian interventions for the capacity of the state and civil society? Does humanitarian assistance strengthen, or weaken, the reconstruction and recovery of national health systems?

Activity 4.2

You are a field worker for an international NGO that prides itself on adherence to humanitarian principles. You are working in eastern DRC, delivering emergency health services to civilians displaced by fierce fighting between government and rebel forces, using tents and a few undamaged buildings. The local government health officer proposes that you use local health clinics to deliver your services. Some of these clinics were badly damaged by the war and the DRC government has secured international funding to rebuild and repair them. He is willing to share this funding with your organization, take part in renovating these clinics, and staff the clinics with available health workers, paid by the DRC government. In return, he would like your organization to offer services from these clinics and provide training to government doctors and nurses to improve their skills.

When preparing your responses, you may wish to consult the *IASC Handbook for Resident Coordinators and Health Coordinators on Emergency Preparedness and Response* (IASC, 2010a).

4.2.1 Do you think a partnership with the government in provision of health services – a government that is actively involved in a conflict – violates international humanitarian norms?

4.2.2 How could you ensure that delivery of humanitarian assistance builds rather than weakens local health system capacity?

4.2.3 What are the advantages and dangers of working with local doctors and nurses to improve their skills?

Conclusions

The international community engages in conflict-affected states for various political and economic reasons, and health is an important component of that engagement. The effectiveness of health responses to crises has improved with the growing evidence base. However, this engagement is not without challenges and contradictions. Health service delivery must navigate an environment with an extremely diverse set of actors – political, humanitarian, and military – working towards ambitious objectives that are not always congruent. While debates remain and too many civilians continue to suffer the effects of violent conflict, the enhanced engagement of the international community and the apparent success in reducing the aggregate impact of war on civilian populations is a hopeful sign for the future. The next chapter will examine the humanitarian system in more detail.

Feedback on activities

Feedback on Activity 4.1

4.1.1 There is no one correct answer. Pages iv–v of the *IASC Civil-Military Guidelines* (IASC, 2008) summarize key issues, and you may have considered that repairing the hospital would be more relevant for NATO interests in 'winning hearts and minds' than for the local population who might be unable to use it if it becomes a target. As the *Guidelines* state, particular caution should be exercised in circumstances where there is a risk that either the motivation for the use of military or civil defence assets or its consequences may be perceived as reflecting political rather than humanitarian considerations.

4.1.2 Whether humanitarian principles should apply to military reconstruction projects is still debated, but you may have argued that they should. It is generally agreed that decisions to accept military assets must be made by humanitarian organizations, not political authorities, and based solely on humanitarian criteria. Military assets should be requested only where there is no comparable civilian alternative and only the use of military assets can meet a critical humanitarian need. The military asset must therefore be unique in nature or timeliness of deployment, and its use should be a last resort.

4.1.3 There are a number of parameters commonly considered. You may have noted that a humanitarian operation using military assets must retain its civilian nature and character. The operation must remain under the overall authority and control of the humanitarian organization responsible for that operation, in this case WHO, whatever the specific command arrangements for the military assets used in making repairs. Additionally, as far as possible, military assets should be unarmed and civilian in appearance.

Feedback on Activity 4.2

4.2.1 You will notice many references to engaging national governments and local stakeholders in the *IASC Handbook* (IASC, 2010a). However, in practice, active partnership with national government authorities is difficult. A particular difficulty you may have considered is that working with government may violate the humanitarian principles of neutrality and independence.

4.2.2 Due to the differing time-frames, priorities and capacities of the humanitarian community and local government, little guidance exists on best practices for such engagement while violence is ongoing. You might consider what you think such guidance and best practices should be, which would still maintain adherence to humanitarian principles.

4.2.3 You may have considered that the major advantage of working with local doctors and nurses is that capacity built is more likely to remain in the country where it is most needed. A disadvantage in the short term might be that staff training can distract from immediate humanitarian priorities (i.e. saving lives) and could be considered a development rather than humanitarian activity.

The humanitarian system

Fiona Campbell and Natasha Howard

Overview

The aim of this chapter is to describe the humanitarian system, focusing on underlying principles, legal framework, and key institutional actors. Concepts from the global health policy literature and policy-making initiatives related to conflict-affected settings are used to frame the current system, ethical issues, and inherent challenges.

Learning outcomes

After completing this chapter you should be able to:

- describe the origins and structure of the humanitarian system, including the main actors relevant to health
- explain core principles and governance mechanisms underpinning humanitarian action
- assess some of the ethical issues and challenges inherent in the system and ongoing reform efforts to support more effective action

Structure of the humanitarian system

...the humanitarian instinct − the urge to help others − is one of the oldest and most noble of human characteristics. It is practiced in many ways in many parts of the world. No single culture or institutional system has the monopoly on humanitarian wisdom. (Mukesh Kapila, 2005)

Defining the humanitarian system and action

While the terms are widely used, there is no agreed definition covering all actions and actors involved in international humanitarian response (Borton, 2009). Here we define the **humanitarian system** as the diverse collective of local, national and international **institutional actors** and networks, with shared goals and associated norms, involved in providing assistance to save lives, alleviate suffering and maintain human dignity during and after human-caused and natural disasters (Harvey et al., 2011).

Humanitarian action can be defined broadly as any action to save lives and alleviate human suffering in crises, particularly when there is an actual or imminent threat to life, health or security. Some distinguish between the actions of a formal international system (e.g. donor governments, UN agencies, the Red Cross and Red Crescent Movement, international non-governmental organizations (INGOs)) and informal system (e.g. affected governments, civil society, military, private sector, affected populations). However, this distinction between formal and informal can give an overly narrow analysis of the humanitarian system and outcomes.

Origins of the humanitarian system

The humanitarian system has evolved over more than a century into what it is today and continues to evolve through ongoing lessons from new humanitarian responses and new actors joining the system (Walker, 2007). It has thus developed, with certain anomalies and irregularities, along four recognizable and often competing political agendas of containment, compassion, change and welfare (Walker, 2007; Walker and Maxwell, 2008).

Containment. While some may argue that humanitarian instinct goes back centuries, most credit the mid-nineteenth century – with its increased globalization through railways and telegraph – as the start of formal international initiatives (Walker, 2007). The initial agenda was primarily one of containment, in which state and state-sponsored religious, commercial and philanthropic actors became involved in mass famine relief and public works efforts from the 1837–8 Indian famine and the 1845–9 Irish famine to the 1920 Sudan famine (Walker, 2007). The language was primarily that of containment, with recipients considered as destitute 'beggars' and 'vagrants', threatening social order and requiring discipline and obedience to colonial authority. It can be argued that state policy is still largely one of containment (though the language has matured), as humanitarian crises often contribute to instability and security challenges for trade and resources (Walker, 2007).

Compassion. Jean-Henri Dunant, whose 1862 book, *A Memory of Solferino*, inspired the creation of the International Committee of the Red Cross (ICRC) and International Red Cross and Red Crescent Movement, is credited with founding modern compassionate humanitarianism (Walker and Maxwell, 2008). This new agenda, rather than countering threats to stability, explicitly aimed to increase moral compassion, alleviate human suffering and promote human dignity and welfare without considering politics or history (Walker, 2007).

Change. In 1919, in response to Allied blockades against Germany and Austria-Hungary, the English activist Eglantine Jebb established the Save the Children Fund (SCF) and the Geneva-based Save the Children Union. SCF was the first transnational humanitarian NGO, and others followed its independent activist model (Walker, 2007). In devising and lobbying successfully for adoption of the Declaration of the Rights of the Child by the League of Nations in 1924 and the Convention on the Rights of the Child by the UN in 1989, SCF promoted the political change agenda, thus challenging containment.

Welfare. After World War II, the Food and Agriculture Organization (FAO) was created in 1945 to strengthen recovery by distributing food surpluses to areas in need. Similarly, 22 US charities organized a mechanism to distribute surplus army food rations to needy families in Europe – thus forming the Cooperative for American Remittances to Europe. By the 1980s, its work and mandate had expanded significantly and its name was changed to Cooperative for Assistance and Relief Everywhere (CARE). The welfare agenda is sometimes described as a soft version of containment, in that it seeks to reduce suffering rather than challenge political or moral realities.

By 1970, the modern international humanitarian system of donor countries, UN system agencies, Red Cross and Red Crescent Movement, major international NGOs, international conventions governing treatment of non-combatants and refugees, human rights conventions, and delivery mechanisms for relief and food aid was in place. However, the large number of actors with differing agendas, collaborating, competing and sometimes undermining each other has created an organic and often chaotic environment rather than the coherent humanitarian system we might wish to see.

International humanitarian system actors

Many diverse actors work within the humanitarian system, some of whom will be familiar from Chapter 4. Actors include those affected by crises and the local, national and international humanitarian workers and institutions involved in providing assistance on their behalf. Actors will vary by context, determined by a range of factors including the nature of the required response (e.g. acute natural disaster, prolonged conflict), the proximity to international responders (e.g. a response in the Balkans will differ from one in Nepal), and political or geographical access (e.g. North Korea traditionally poses political access challenges for humanitarian initiatives, while parts of Afghanistan pose physical access challenges).

International actors with a major role in humanitarian action include the UN system agencies, (e.g. World Health Organization (WHO), FAO, UN High Commissioner for Refugees (UNHCR)); bilateral and multilateral donors (e.g. Department for International Development (DFID), European Commission); INGOs and faith-based organizations (e.g. Médecins Sans Frontières, Médecins du Monde, World Vision); the International Federation of the Red Cross and Red Crescent Movement (IFRC); the military; and the private sector. We look at some of these actors in more detail below.

UN agencies. Agencies within the UN that play a key role in humanitarian action include those with a specialist mandate (e.g. WHO and health), those focused on specific groups (e.g. UNICEF and children, UNHCR and internally displaced persons) respectively, and those delivering particular aspects of relief (e.g. the World Food Programme and basic food commodities). WHO, UNICEF and UNHCR are lead agencies for health. Both WHO and UNICEF have dedicated units for humanitarian issues (e.g. WHO/Health Action in Crisis department). UNHCR is mandated to lead and coordinate international action to protect and support refugees and displaced populations.

The UN Office for the Coordination of Humanitarian Affairs (OCHA) was established in 1998 to mobilize and coordinate humanitarian assistance delivered by international and national partners. The head of OCHA is the Under-Secretary-General for Humanitarian Affairs and the Emergency Relief Coordinator. OCHA usually becomes involved when a multi-sectoral international response is required. At country level, coordination of relief efforts is managed by the UN Humanitarian Coordinator (see the subsection on *coordination mechanisms* on page 51 for more).

International donors. The number of **international donors** – bilateral and multilateral donors supporting international humanitarian responses – has nearly doubled in recent years. Government donors vary in the size and scope of the departments responsible for overseeing their humanitarian engagement and contributions. In 2008, over 100 governments reported humanitarian contributions, with the three largest humanitarian donors in total funds being the USA (US$4.4 billion), the European institutions (US$1.6 billion) and the UK (US$1 billion) (ALNAP, 2010). While figures vary from year to year, these three have been key donors over many years and active in supporting humanitarian health action (Global Humanitarian Assistance, 2011). The UK, the Netherlands, Norway, Sweden, Canada and Ireland have been proactive in supporting humanitarian reform (ALNAP, 2010). The current dominance of Western donors appears to be declining due to growing humanitarian contributions by countries such as Saudi Arabia, Kuwait, China, and India (Binder et al., 2010).

The International Red Cross and Red Crescent Movement consists of several legally independent organizations, linked through common principles, objectives, symbols and governance mechanisms. The ICRC, the International Federation of Red Cross and Red Crescent Societies (IFRC) and 186 national Red Cross and Red Crescent societies, make up the world's largest independent humanitarian network. The Movement's seven principles of humanity, impartiality, neutrality, independence, voluntary service, unity and universality were added to official statutes in 1986. The ICRC is a private association credited with initiating modern international humanitarian law (IHL) and has a special mandate through the Geneva Conventions to protect and assist victims of armed conflict and develop, implement and promote IHL, making it unique among humanitarian actors.

Non-governmental organizations are legally-constituted associations, operating independently of governments with a social or sociopolitical agenda, and normally non-profit. A large number of NGOs, both national and international, are involved in humanitarian action. An estimated 250 organizations, multilateral federations and their national affiliates, make up the global humanitarian NGO community. Some have built up years of experience, responding to a range of disasters and conflicts, while others may form for a particular response. Six large international NGOs (INGOs) dominate: CARE, Catholic Relief Services, Médecins Sans Frontières, Oxfam, Save the Children International, and World Vision International (ALNAP, 2010). Several smaller INGOs focus on humanitarian health action, including Merlin, International Refugee Committee (IRC) and Médecins du Monde. INGOs are not homogeneous, and distinctions have been drawn between the *Dunantist* humanitarianism of European NGOs, which aim to remain disconnected from state interests, and the *Wilsonian* humanitarianism of US NGOs, whose actions are considered as serving the same purposes as government activities.

The *Steering Committee for Humanitarian Response* (SCHR), created in 1972, is an alliance of chief executive officers representing nine humanitarian networks and agencies (i.e. Care International, Caritas International, ICRC, IFRC, International Save the Children Alliance, Lutheran World Federation, Oxfam, World Council of Churches, and World Vision International). In 1994, it founded the *Code of Conduct for International Red Cross and Red Crescent Movement and NGOs in Disaster Relief*. In 1997, with the US-based InterAction NGO consortium, it initiated the *Sphere Project* to develop a set of minimum standards, improve quality and increase accountability in humanitarian assistance.

National NGOs and **community-based organizations** (CBOs) have long been vital in humanitarian response and many INGOs work through national or community-level partners during humanitarian operations. Their diversity makes it difficult to characterize the range of competences and approaches. Community actors are generally closest to the emergency, can act fastest, and may be able to gain access where international agencies cannot. They can provide local knowledge to explain local tensions and help ensure community needs are addressed (GHWA et al., 2011). However, they may also have their own agendas and biases, which are important to acknowledge.

National governments are more frequently responding to crises without external assistance and even rejecting offers of help (ALNAP, 2010). The relationship between humanitarian agencies and host governments can be sensitive, especially in conflict settings. However, international efforts have not always taken national capacity and systems into consideration, and ensuring that national health systems are not undermined is important even during conflict.

Non-humanitarian system actors

Some actors are often involved in humanitarian responses (e.g. private sector, military), but not considered part of the humanitarian system, as they are not bound by the humanitarian principles (see the subsection on *humanitarian principles* below).

Private sector humanitarian responses may be both commercial and altruistic. Large international firms have provided support in response to disasters, often pro bono, with logistics and telecommunications. Local private firms may be early and important responders. While some recommend increased engagement with the private sector and usage of its resources and expertise, reticence continues about engaging fully with the 'for-profit' sector and private sector actors may be excluded from extensive participation within the wider humanitarian system (DFID, 2011).

The military may work beside humanitarian agencies in peace-keeping, or peace enforcement, missions. As part of this role, there is a growing trend for military humanitarian and development activities, often in furtherance of a 'hearts and minds' campaign to gain acceptance among affected populations. The military role in humanitarian activity is contentious in blurring the lines between security strategies and humanitarian principles of neutrality and impartiality. While in some contexts the military may be the only agency with the expertise and assets to provide a timely response, engagement with the military has potential repercussions for accessing populations and the safety of humanitarian workers (Global Humanitarian Assistance, 2011).

Activity 5 .1

Choose a recent conflict with a humanitarian response that was covered by international media.

5.1.1 Which humanitarian actors received the most media attention, and do you think this reflected the true nature of the humanitarian response?
5.1.2 Which other actors are likely to have played a significant role, and why might their efforts have been given less attention?

Humanitarian governance

Humanitarian principles

The core humanitarian principles guiding humanitarian action are humanity, impartiality, independence and neutrality – though the last is not practiced by all actors. *Humanity* signifies that all human beings are equal in dignity and rights, thus all human life and health should be respected and protected and human suffering reduced. *Impartiality* signifies that humanitarian assistance must be provided solely according to need, without distinction by nationality, ethnicity, social class, religion, gender, or politics.

Independence signifies that humanitarian action must be autonomous with respect to political, economic, military or other objectives. *Neutrality* signifies that humanitarian actors cannot take sides in conflicts or engage in controversies concerning politics, ethnicity, religion or ideology (OCHA, 2010).

These principles have been adopted by over 400 organizations globally and formally endorsed in two UN General Assembly resolutions. Resolution A/46/182 included neutrality and impartiality and led to the creation of the Department of Humanitarian Affairs, later OCHA. Resolution A/58/114 included independence, further emphasized coordinated humanitarian action, and led to development of the Emergency Relief Coordinator role. However, implementing humanitarian principles can be challenging.

The fourth principle of neutrality is perhaps the most contentious. It is included in the International Red Cross and Red Crescent Movement statutes and Resolution 46/182 for UN system agencies, but is not part of the *Code of Conduct for International Red Cross and Red Crescent Movement and NGOs in Disaster Relief* (1994) to which all SCHR members are signatories. Its current usage among many agencies is provision of humanitarian assistance in an impartial and independent manner, as political neutrality would preclude lobbying on social justice and human rights initiatives. Agencies with multiple mandates, combining humanitarian and longer-term development aims, may find neutrality difficult.

International humanitarian law

International humanitarian law, or *jus in bello*, regulates the conduct of armed conflict and treatment of non-combatants. Along with *jus ad bellum*, concerning acceptable justifications for engaging in war, it forms a body of public international law sometimes called the *laws of war*. IHL consists of the Hague Conventions of 1899 and 1907, defining responsibilities and acceptable actions of belligerent nations, and the Geneva Conventions, defining acceptable treatment of civilians and former combatants, plus subsequent treaties, customary international law and case law. The four Geneva Conventions and three associated protocols are as follows:

* *First Geneva Convention for the Amelioration of the Condition of the Wounded and Sick in Armed Forces in the Field*, adopted in 1864 and last revised in 1949;
* *Second Geneva Convention for the Amelioration of the Condition of Wounded, Sick and Shipwrecked Members of Armed Forces at Sea* (1949) to succeed the 1907 Hague Convention X;
* *Third Geneva Convention relative to the Treatment of Prisoners of War*, adopted in 1929 and last revised in 1949;
* *Fourth Geneva Convention relative to the Protection of Civilian Persons in Time of War* (1949), partly based on the 1907 Hague Convention IV;
* Protocol I (1977), relating to protection of victims of international armed conflicts, ratified by approximately 170 countries;
* Protocol II (1977), relating to protection of victims of non-international armed conflicts, ratified by approximately 165 countries;
* Protocol III (2005), relating to adoption of an additional distinctive emblem, ratified by approximately 17 countries.

IHL aims to protect non-combatants, including prisoners of war, civilian and displaced populations, and humanitarian workers (ICRC, 2004). Serious violations of the Hague

Conventions, and subsequent London Charter and Nuremburg principles, are categorized as war crimes, crimes against peace, or crimes against humanity.

Coordination mechanisms

Given the number of actors engaged in humanitarian interventions, the international humanitarian community created coordination mechanisms to ensure a more effective professional humanitarian response. Key mechanisms include the **cluster approach** and the consolidated appeals process.

The cluster approach, established during humanitarian reforms in 2005, has now been rolled out in over 30 countries (e.g. DRC, Libya). Different UN agencies are designated global **cluster** leads, responsible for providing an effective inter-agency response within 11 areas of humanitarian response (Figure 5.1). These include food security (FAO/WFP), nutrition (UNICEF), camp coordination (UNHCR), logistics (WFP), protection (UNHCR), emergency shelter (UNHCR/IFRC), emergency telecommunications (WFP), education (UNICEF/SCF), water sanitation and hygiene (UNICEF), health (WHO) and early recovery (UNDP). At the global level, lead agencies establish operational standards. At the national and field levels they are expected to coordinate the responses of multinational actors. Although there are advantages to the same agency leading at international, national and field levels, sometimes NGOs have successfully taken on a cluster co-stewardship role at national and sub-national levels. It is important to note existing exceptions to the Cluster approach (e.g. refugee responses are always led by UNHCR). Humanitarian situations can occur in which the responsible government is strong enough not to require it or chooses not to implement the Cluster approach (e.g. Sri Lanka, Syria, Afghanistan).

The *Global Health Cluster* (GHC) is under WHO leadership and includes more than 30 international humanitarian health organizations. Priorities include developing country-level capacity to design, implement and monitor evidence-based health responses; ensure human and material resources are available to country clusters; identify health priorities in humanitarian settings and coordinate actions at the global level to address them; and monitor the effectiveness of the health cluster at the global and country levels. At global level, cluster partners are involved in development and dissemination of cluster tools, guidelines, and common position papers, and training health cluster coordinators. Position papers, to support country-level decision-making, have included removal of user fees in emergencies and civil–military cooperation. At country level, health cluster partners coordinate information gathering, analysis, and prioritization of interventions. Challenges with the approach include the number of agencies involved at country level (e.g. over 300 in Haiti), making coordinated action almost impossible (Doull, 2011).

In December 2011, after analysing leadership and coordination challenges, the IASC agreed a set of actions to substantively improve the current humanitarian response model. As part of the IASC Principles Transformative Agenda 2012, a number of changes are being made to the Cluster approach (see the IASC website for the latest information). The consolidated appeals process (CAP) is another tool to ensure a coordinated and effective response to humanitarian crises. The CAP, led by OCHA, is used by humanitarian actors to assess population needs; determine and plan appropriate evidence-based responses; coordinate how various agencies will contribute to the overall response; and seek money from donors to support these activities. Multiple iterations of the CAP are often released; with the first flash appeal being quickly prepared to mobilize resources and subsequent appeals containing more detail on needs, responses and costs.

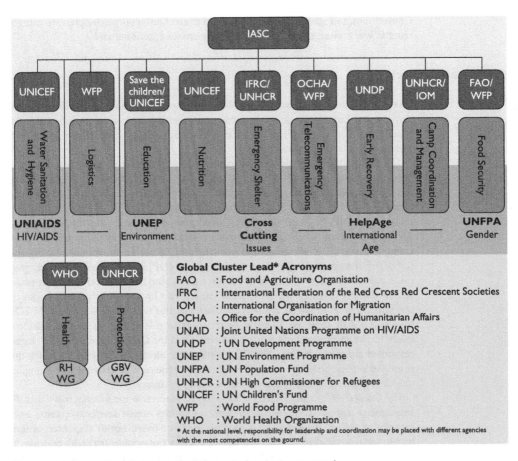

Figure 5.1 Humanitarian coordination through the cluster approach
Source: MISP online training course (RHRC, 2011).

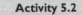 **Activity 5.2**

Consider the same humanitarian response as in Activity 5.1 or another and reflect on the four principles of humanitarian action.

5.2.1 Why are these principles important in the context you have chosen?
5.2.2 What challenges do you see in upholding these principles in your chosen context?

Humanitarian reform

Ethical norms

Two opposing normative ethical approaches underpin humanitarian responses and approaches to reform. In *moral absolutism*, actions are either right or wrong in themselves, regardless of context or outcome. Thus, there is a moral imperative to act and longer-term outcomes are of lesser consequence. In *utilitarianism*, a consequentialist ethical approach, the longer-term outcome matters most and short-term gains may be sacrificed to achieve this. Ethical norms underpinning agency engagement affect the nature of assistance provided (Slim, 1997). European humanitarian NGOs are seen to favour moral absolutist approaches, while UK and US agencies are considered to favour a utilitarian emphasis on addressing the underlying causes of crises. In practice, this distinction may not be apparent (Sondorp, 2011).

All interventions should be considered in terms of their potential to cause unwanted negative outcomes as well as intended good. Provision of humanitarian assistance during conflict can, if poorly conceived or managed, support continued conflict and cause harm. There are five ways in which humanitarian action can cause harm: (i) diversion of resources to support armies, such as through theft; (ii) affecting markets potentially supporting the war; (iii) reinforcing tensions between groups; (iv) freeing local resources to support the conflict; and (v) providing legitimacy for the actions or agendas of those seeking conflict (Anderson, 1999). Safeguarding against potential unintended harm is an ethical imperative in any humanitarian response or reform effort.

Humanitarian accountability

In 2009, more than two-thirds of all humanitarian assistance went to conflict-affected and post-conflict states (Global Humanitarian Assistance, 2011). How the humanitarian system responds to conflict is thus a critical marker of overall system performance. The international humanitarian response for 2010 was estimated at US$16.7 billion (Global Humanitarian Assistance, 2011). Humanitarian engagement is a huge enterprise and requires effective mechanisms to ensure it delivers on its commitments. Efforts to promote quality and effectiveness rely on agency choice and normative influence as no overall body monitors adherence to codes and standards.

Attempts by the humanitarian community to promote good practice include codes and guidelines such as the 1994 *Code of Conduct for International Red Cross and Red Crescent Movement and NGOs in Disaster Relief*, the 1997 Sphere Project, the 1997 Active Learning Network for Accountability and Performance in Humanitarian Action (ALNAP), and the 2003 Humanitarian Accountability Partnership (HAP) International and Good Humanitarian Donorship (GHD) initiatives (DFID, 2011).

The *Code of Conduct*, discussed earlier in this chapter, has been particularly influential and is frequently quoted by agencies wishing to demonstrate their humanitarian credentials (IFRC and ICRC, 1996).

The *Sphere Project* developed a set of minimum standards for humanitarian response against which programmes can be assessed across sectors (e.g. WASH promotion; food security and nutrition; shelter, settlement and non-food items; health action) and eight cross-cutting themes (children, gender, older people, disabilities, psychosocial support, HIV, environment, disaster risk reduction). The *Sphere Handbook*, revised in 2011, has become a ubiquitous guide for humanitarian response (Sphere, 2011).

ALNAP, also established following the multi-agency evaluation of the Rwanda genocide, is a network of donors, UN, Red Cross and Red Crescent societies, NGOs and academics, aiming to improve quality and accountability.

HAP International is a multi-agency self-regulatory body established to promote accountability to persons affected by crises by those acting on their behalf. It provides accreditation standards and accountability framework by which humanitarian agencies can be certified according to the quality and accountability of their work (Humanitarian Accountability Partnership, 2010).

The *GHD initiative* is an informal donor network facilitating collective good practice, based on the *Principles and Good Practice of Good Humanitarian Donorship*, developed by founders Australia, Belgium, Canada, Denmark, the European Commission, Finland, France, Germany, Ireland, Japan, Luxemburg, the Netherlands, Norway, Sweden, Switzerland, the UK, and the US. The initiative aims to enhance the coherence and effectiveness of donor action and accountability to beneficiaries, implementing organizations and domestic constituencies in funding, coordination, follow-up and evaluation.

Humanitarian reform

The perceived failure of the international response in Sudan in 2004 prompted a major review of the humanitarian system. This focused on improving the timeliness and effectiveness of collective action, and the reforms that followed aimed to improve the consistency and quality of humanitarian services. Reforms covered three main elements: (i) improving response capacity through the cluster approach discussed above; (ii) improving humanitarian coordination; and (iii) improving the predictability of humanitarian financing through a Central Emergency Relief Fund (CERF).

The effectiveness of the *cluster approach* has been variable. While evaluations have pointed to increased coverage, better identification of gaps and less duplication of efforts, a number of challenges remain regarding impact on national and local ownership and capacities (Steets et al., 2010).

Coordination through the *humanitarian coordinators system* has also had mixed success. Humanitarian coordinators often do not have a strong humanitarian background, being chosen from a general pool of UN staff and at times fulfilling multiple roles. Thus success has depended on the individual in post and their particular experience and interest (Waldman, 2011).

The third area of reform is promotion of predictable rapid-response financing through *CERF* that will also address underfunded emergencies. CERF has performed reasonably well since inception. However, challenges include increasing bureaucracy in disbursement of funds and dissatisfaction, particularly among NGOs, with disbursements through UN agencies (Waldman, 2011). Thus, reforms remain a work in progress, not yet having resulted in a system that meets current and future challenges.

Activity 5.3

Efforts to manage growth, improve performance and increase professionalism within the humanitarian system have contributed a growing number of standards (e.g. Sphere, ALNAP), coordination (e.g. the cluster approach), and accountability mechanisms (e.g. the *Code of Conduct*).

5.2.1 Review the current edition of the ALNAP *State of the Humanitarian System* report (Harvey et al., 2011), available online, and identify some potential effects of current funding and human resource levels.

5.2.2 What are some pros and cons of coordination mechanisms such as the cluster approach?

Conclusions

This chapter summarizes the humanitarian system, including origins, main humanitarian actors relevant to health, principles, governance mechanisms and ethical norms underpinning humanitarian action, and accountability and reform challenges inherent in the system. The next chapters will address humanitarian health interventions.

Feedback on activities

Feedback on Activity 5.1

Your response will depend on the conflict you have chosen and your information sources. Conflicts with a large international response may receive extensive global media coverage.

5.1.1 Global media coverage is likely to highlight the role of international actors, particularly those from the country to which the report is being distributed. In many cases, the media may be used by international actors to gain publicity for their actions in the hope of raising funds for their agency or the crisis more generally.

5.1.2 The role of national actors in the response may not have featured so prominently in global media reports. However, they will have been there and many international agencies are likely to have partnered with local actors with the aim of increasing local access and acceptability. The question why local actors might have been given less attention is a complex one. While international humanitarian agencies have become increasingly transnational in scope, financing and accountability are still largely Northern (i.e. European, North American). How can partnership work best given these realities? (For example, are such partnerships contractual, control-based and led by local knowledge?) Consider how the humanitarian system could move beyond the traditionally Northern, establishment roots of many of its actors.

Feedback on Activity 5.2

While your answers will depend on the conflict chosen, certain themes are likely to emerge.

5.2.1 Actors will be expected to ensure that they preserve humanity and impartiality. Independence can be challenged by available funding or compromises necessary to gain access to affected populations. Neutrality has become less widely held, partly as a consequence of the atrocities committed in the Balkans and Rwanda conflicts and also because contemporary asymmetric conflicts, with their non-traditional combatants, mean its effectiveness in ensuring the safety of humanitarian actors is significantly reduced.

5.2.2 If you chose a context in which the international community is involved in military action, you may have considered challenges to impartiality and independence and how to ensure that humanitarian action is not seen as furthering any wider political or military agenda. If you chose a 'network' or civil conflict, in which one side of the conflict may be the government, you would have considered how providing health care or health system support might be viewed as siding with the government (e.g. is it viewed as purely technical or as supporting a wider state-building agenda?). Would health system support undermine neutrality or can humanitarian actors provide support to both government and non-government sides (e.g. to both Afghan government and the Taliban in Afghanistan)?

Feedback on Activity 5.3

5.3.1 Figures indicate approximately 210,800 acute and post-acute crisis workers in the field in 2008, up 6% annually in the previous 10 years. Funding estimates lie in the range US$6.6–18 billion for the same year. Potential effects you may have identified include the increased professionalization of the system and actors, increased formalization of structures and reduced ability to tailor responses to individual contexts, increased politicization and accountability to donor agendas.

5.3.2 As Walker (2007) notes: 'Everyone wants coordination; no one wants to be coordinated.' While the positive aspects of coordination may be obvious (e.g. greater collective influence, the ability to detect and fill gaps, increased efficiency), it comes at the price of some loss of independence.

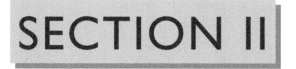

SECTION II

Humanitarian health interventions

Initial assessment and priority setting 6

Nadine Ezard and Chris Lewis

Overview

This aim of this chapter is to provide an overview of objectives and approaches in initial humanitarian health assessment, focusing on identifying intervention priorities to reduce avoidable mortality, morbidity and suffering in conflict. Concepts from programme management and fieldwork in conflict-affected settings are used.

Learning outcomes

After completing this chapter you should be able to:

* explain initial assessment and types of humanitarian health assessment
* identify data collection needs in humanitarian health assessments
* describe data collection methods and interpretation for prioritizing intervention areas

What is humanitarian assessment?

Defining assessment

Initial humanitarian assessments, also called needs assessments, are a systematic way of gathering and analysing relevant information to determine implementation approaches based on available data and response capacity. Assessing the context, status and magnitude of a crisis is considered an essential part of humanitarian response. Large-scale crises attract a multitude of actors, from a range of sectors, with a range of capacities and institutional mandates. Due to humanitarian reforms, increasing efforts are made to formalize and coordinate initial assessments across agencies and sectors.

Assessment aims

Initial assessments aim to identify unmet population needs and gaps in the information needed to define and measure needs. Each actor needs information to decide whether or not to intervene, guide the nature and scale of intervention, prioritize resource allocation, and inform programme design. Some agencies choose to identify and address the needs of the most vulnerable, while others focus on the most important causes of avoidable illness and death for the majority of the affected population (Darcy and Hofman, 2003).

The primary reason for initial assessment, as defined here, is to identify key priorities for action. Assessment is the first stage of a programme planning cycle, followed by programme design, implementation, monitoring and evaluation (see Chapter 10).

Assessment types

Initial assessment allows rapid analysis of known influences on population health and survival, including protection, shelter, water, sanitation, nutrition, and health. The different types of initial humanitarian assessment are as follows (IASC, 2011a):

- *Coordinated assessment.* Assessment is planned and conducted by a partnership of humanitarian actors and results shared to help the broader humanitarian community identify population needs.
- *Harmonized assessment.* Data collection, processing and analysis are undertaken separately, but data are sufficiently comparable, due to use of common operational data sets, key indicators, and geographical and temporal synchronization, to be compiled in a single database and used in shared analysis.
- *Joint assessment.* Data collection, processing and analysis form a single process among agencies within and between sectors and leads to a single report (also called *common assessment*).
- *Individual agency assessment.* An assessment by an individual agency, chiefly to inform programme design. Assessment orientation may be influenced by the agency's capacities, resources, and motivations.
- *Multi-sectoral assessment.* This type brings sectors together for joint assessment, using one agreed methodology, so that data collection, processing, and analysis are aligned into a single process. A multi-sectoral assessment should identify the overall impact of the crisis and priority needs using a mixture of secondary and primary data. Following operational division of humanitarian response into clusters (see Chapter 5), increasingly agencies are using standard multi-sectoral assessment tools for initial assessments, followed by in-depth health sector assessments (see Table 6.1 for phasing of assessments).
- *Health sector assessment.* In-depth assessment of health sector agencies and health systems.
- *Sub-sectoral or cross-sectoral assessment.* Designed to assess specific areas relevant to population health (e.g. **gender-based violence**, mental health and psychosocial support, reproductive health, and substance use), these usually follow from broader multi-sectoral assessments and health sector assessments, but may be conducted earlier of specific risks are identified.

Assessment approaches

Assessment approaches vary. They may be limited to assessing current status or go further to assess humanitarian needs, unmet needs, or future hazards. A good assessment should enable prioritization of those interventions that maximize impact while ensuring incremental restoration of population self-sufficiency. However, humanitarian

Table 6.1 Phased approach to humanitarian assessment in an acute onset emergency

Timing	Phase 0 Before	Phase 1 72 hours	Phase 2 Week 1–2	Phase 3 Week 3+	Phase 4 2nd month +
Assessment type	**Assessment preparedness**	**Initial assessment**	**Rapid assessment** More than one sector	**In-depth assessment** Single sector	**In-depth assessment** Single sector with early recovery considerations
Assessment purpose	Preparedness planning and gathering pre-crisis data	Estimate scale and severity of the event. Locate affected populations. Inform initial response decisions. Inform phase 2 rapid assessments	Inform initial planning of humanitarian response, highlighting priority actions. Define focus for following in-depth assessments. Establish baseline for monitoring	Analyse situation and trends. Adjust ongoing response. Inform detailed planning for relief/early recovery. Establish baseline for monitoring	Analyse situation and trends. Inform phase-out of life-sustaining activities. Inform detailed planning for relief to early recovery transition. Feed into performance monitoring
Data sources		Mostly secondary sources (e.g. published documents, agency reports, initial field reports, media, pre-crisis reports, satellite imagery, pre-crisis surveys and health surveillance data). *Primary data:* direct observation from quick field visits, information from funding monitoring/reporting systems	Various secondary sources. *Primary data:* As phase 1, complemented by purposive site visits, community/key informant interviews. Unit of measurement for site visits is community (e.g. village, camp) or institution (e.g. school, health facility). Detailed assessment (e.g. mortality, malnutrition survey) may be initiated	Various secondary sources. *Primary data:* As in phase 2, but purposive and representative methods used for site visits. New data from (re-)established monitoring systems. Unit of measurement as in phase 2, plus household and individual	As in phase 3

Source: Adapted from IASC (2011a).

assessments are often done badly due to time limitations; operational, geographical, and security constraints; competing motivations and capacities of intervening agencies; complexity of assessment tools; need for situation-specific information; and the imperative for rapid response.

A phased approach is usually taken with an initial multi-sectoral assessment in the first few hours or days of an acute onset emergency, and more detailed sectoral, sub-sectoral or single-issue assessments in the days or weeks following. Reassessments are also necessary as the situation stabilizes or changes.

Table 6.1 shows a schema for stepwise phasing of different types of assessments in a hypothetical acute onset emergency. Phase 0 focuses on assessment preparedness and gathering pre-crisis data. Phase 1 and 2 aim for a broad overview to inform initial planning and highlight priority actions. Most initial information will be collected from a review of the published literature and agency documents and secondary data from health facilities or other services if available. From week 3 onwards, assessments become narrower – focusing on specific sectors and sub-sectors – using purposively selected primary data and secondary data to analyse trends (e.g. most important causes of morbidity and mortality, most affected groups) to inform planning for priorities and recovery activities. Health assessments may be conducted while initial activities are completed (e.g. erecting temporary shelters, delivering emergency food rations, conducting measles vaccination campaigns). The situation may not have stabilized yet, amidst ongoing population fluctuations and security concerns.

The initial phase of an acute crisis is often confusing, with contradictory information, multiple competing needs, difficult operating environments, instability, ongoing population movement, and limited resources – notably people and transport – required for assessment. Thus, multi-sector assessments help determine the scale of the crisis, locate the populations most affected, and identify priorities for action. Coordination and timely information sharing can maximize use of available resources, speed data collection, build an overall picture of the situation, and avoid duplication of efforts.

Case study

Côte d'Ivoire, January 2011 (ACP, 2011). Côte d'Ivoire is experiencing escalating violence, particularly in the West of the country and around the largest city, Abidjan, in the wake of contested national elections on 28 November 2010. Reports suggest around 250 deaths and thousands injured. Fear of violence has led to major population movements within the country and to neighbouring countries – an estimated 30,000 have fled to Liberia, 17,000 are internally displaced in camps, and 75,000 are living with host families in the West of the country amid continued military clashes. The Internally displaced population is reported to have limited access to basic services and serious protection concerns, particularly women and children. Identification of humanitarian needs and relief interventions in Côte d'Ivoire is made difficult by the deteriorating security situation and movement restrictions for international agencies, both non-governmental and UN. Many expatriate personnel have been evacuated. Little is known about the precise situation in the West of the country as few recent assessments have been conducted. Pre-crisis information includes the following:

- This current outbreak of violence and population movement occurs in the context of prolonged crisis. The country is one of the world's 20 poorest. The civil war of 2002–4 killed thousands, displaced hundreds of thousands, destroyed infrastructure and services, and widened the gap between rural and urban poverty.
- Most of the country's poor are small-scale famers, with 75% of the rural population affected by poverty. The West is classified as 'food insecure' and chronic malnutrition has risen to critical levels (around 45% in 2009).
- Health services and infrastructure are poor. Measles immunization coverage is estimated at 63% (among children aged 12–24 months) and there are 1.4 physicians per 100,000 population.
- Nationally, 56% of the population lives more than 5 kilometres from a health facility. Access to health care in the West is particularly constrained, with most public services closed during the conflict and continuously hampered by disparities in health worker distribution, insufficient financial resources and equipment, insufficient number of health centres, and high cost of services.
- Prevalence of HIV infection among adults aged 15–49 years is 4.7%.
- The main causes of death among children under 5 years are malaria (21%), pneumonia (17%) and diarrhoea (13%).
- Recent outbreaks reported include cholera, which is considered endemic with peak incidence during the wet season (May–June); measles (2010); and yellow fever, associated with disrupted vaccination programmes and movement of non-immune populations into transmission areas (most recently reported in November 2010).

Activity 6.1

Imagine you are the medical officer for a humanitarian NGO. Using the case study, what type of assessment would you recommend if your NGO gains access to the West of the country?

Data needs

Health assessment data needs

Initial assessment requires sufficient reliable information in the shortest possible time; assessments that take too long, even if they collect perfect data, are not useful. Equally, incomplete or badly collected data are misleading, and resulting errors could cause avoidable death or suffering. Prioritization of data needs and activities is key to good assessment.

Community participation in assessing needs is essential. Effective assessment is people-centred and socially inclusive, using and strengthening existing capacities. The degree of participation – from consultation to active management – may depend on the life-threatening urgency of the crisis and local capacity. Necessary data include context, health status, risk factors, and health system status.

Context

Socioeconomics and politics

Affected populations should be described by geographic area, with a brief summary of cultural, economic, physical, political, and social-structural issues to contextualize assessment. Security and protection risks should be outlined. Attempts to understand population diversity (e.g. age, gender, religion, ethnicity, community power relations and divisions) should be included. Some description of existing coping and social-support mechanisms can be important. Many contextual features may have been identified during initial rapid assessment and do not need to be repeated.

Knowledge of pre-crisis health conditions affecting the population, and main health problems in the new environment if displaced, can identify key diseases of public health importance and population health risks. Health assessment should be guided by knowledge of pre-conflict disease **epidemiology** in the affected population, which depends on:

- urban or rural setting
- high or low-income setting
- population demographics, particularly age and sex breakdown
- food security and presence or absence of famine

Pre-crisis infectious disease burden may be particularly important among low-income and young populations. Knowledge of disease seasonality and past disease outbreaks helps predict future health hazards (e.g. acute respiratory infections with impending winter, malaria with impending wet season). Pre-crisis burden of chronic and non-infectious diseases may be important among ageing and high-income and high-life-expectancy populations as conflict may interrupt treatment or exacerbate poor outcomes. Populations from high-income settings may have had good pre-conflict health care coverage.

Knowledge of context may help identify or predict some underlying causes of excess mortality and morbidity, most-affected groups, risk and protective factors, and population vulnerability and resilience. Contextual assessment should briefly describe the pre-crisis health infrastructure and surveillance system and how crisis affected them.

Population size and demographics

The size of the affected population should be defined and disaggregated by age and sex at least. These data are important for assessing the magnitude of the crisis and to calculate mortality and mobility indicators. Population data are easier to obtain in closed settings (e.g. camps) than in open or diffuse settings and can be sensitive and political, particularly if linked to resource allocation. Data are required on: total population, male to female sex ratio, percentages of specific groups (e.g. those under age 5, over age 60, pregnant and lactating), and if possible the demographic pyramid. Expanded data can describe the population by narrower age ranges or other group features (e.g. wealth, social status, legal status, ethnicity, religion). Data disaggregated to this detail may be difficult to obtain in an acute phase response or a small population. Table 6.2 provides data estimations often used in developing countries in the absence of other data.

Table 6.2 Estimated population by age group: example for developing country

Age group (years)	Proportion (%)
0–4	16
5–14	27
15–29	27
30–44	16
≥ 45	14
Pregnant women as proportion of the population	4

Source: Médecins Sans Frontières (2006).

Health status

Mortality data

In conflict-affected, resource-poor settings, most deaths are due to respiratory infections, diarrhoea, malaria (where endemic), measles and neonatal causes. Over half of deaths among children under age 5 (around 53%) have under-nutrition as an underlying cause. Mortality data should be collected on common conditions, noting any unusual or unexpected causes of death. Mortality indicators include:

- *Crude and under-5 mortality* (number of deaths per 10,000 population/day in acute crises and per 1,000 population per month as the situation stabilizes);
- *Infant and maternal mortality* (important but unlikely to be common enough to provide a stable estimate, particularly in small populations over short time-frames);
- *Proportional mortality* (percentage of deaths due to each of the most common diseases, usually expressed among all ages and those under 5 years old);
- *Disease-specific mortality rate* (number of deaths due to a specific disease per person per unit of time, e.g. number of diarrhoea deaths among children under 5 per thousand children under 5 per week);
- *Case fatality rate* (which, for infectious disease outbreaks, effective intervention usually keeps below accepted thresholds (Sphere, 2011) of 1% in the case of cholera, *Shigella* dysentery or typhoid, 5% for measles or severe malaria, or 5–15% for meningococcal meningitis).

Morbidity data

Data should be collected on most common causes of illness, including:

- *proportional morbidity* (percentage of all reported cases due to each of the most common diseases over a specified time period, usually presented for all ages and children under age 5, and useful when population size is not known or rapidly changing);
- *incidence* (number of new cases per population per unit of time, e.g. number of confirmed malaria cases per thousand population per week);

- *prevalence* (percentage of population with a specific disease or outcome at a speci-fied time-point).

Risk factors for ill health

Survival needs

Core needs for population survival include access to an adequate quantity and quality of food, water, sanitation, shelter and essential non-food items (e.g. blankets, cooking fuel). Table 6.3 provides consensus minimum standards for key survival needs. Cross-referencing other sectoral assessments can provide detail on food security, water, sanitation and hygiene, shelter, and non-food needs, responses, and gaps. The physical environment should be reviewed for disease hazards in or nearby settlements, such as vectors (e.g. rats, flies, mosquitoes) and upcoming seasonal changes (see Chapter 8). Urgency and severity should guide decisions on the level of detail required and appro-priate standards for the health assessment.

Vaccination coverage

Estimating measles vaccination coverage among children 9 months to 15 years is part of initial assessment to determine the risk of outbreaks. In acute-onset crises where pre-conflict coverage is known to be high, further investigation is not warranted. However, measles is highly infectious and can spread rapidly in high population densi-ties. In developing countries, case fatality rates are usually less than 5%, but have been known to be higher than 30% in populations with significant malnutrition and poor access to health care. Areas of low vaccination coverage for diphtheria or pertussis are at risk of vaccine-preventable disease outbreaks.

Table 6.3 Sphere minimum standards for humanitarian response

Survival need	Minimum standard
Food	• 2,100 kilocalories per person per day • 10% of total energy provided by protein • 17% of total energy provided by fat • adequate micronutrient intake
Water	• 15 litres of safe water per person per day • accessible within 500 metres and 30-minute wait • two 10–20 litre water containers per household
Sanitation	• One latrine for 20 persons • One bar of laundry and personal soap per person per month
Shelter	• 3.5 square metres of space per person in shelters • 30 square metres per person surface area of overall site (for camps)

Source: Sphere (2011).

Health system analysis

Initial assessment may also look at health system functionality and disruption caused by conflict. The health system is composed of several interrelated components or 'building blocks'. For example, health staff may be working, but services collapse due to lack of medicines or funding. Health system functionality should be assessed at central, regional and local levels, in collaboration with local health authorities.

Important building blocks include health services, health information, disease outbreak early warning systems, health workforce, medical supplies and equipment, leadership and governance, and health financing. Initial assessment may identify information gaps for subsequent in-depth assessment (Pavignani and Colombo, 2009: Module 12).

Health service resources

Assessment should include a review of service coverage, access and usage. A formal health facility assessment may be indicated in the future. Table 6.4 provides example minimum standards for aspects of health service provision, though conclusions regarding needs should be guided by local context.

Table 6.4 Sphere minimum standards for clinical care provision in humanitarian crises

Indicator	Minimum standard
Ratio of functioning health facility/population	1 basic health unit (primary health facility)/ 10,000 population 1 health centre/50,000 population 1 district or rural hospital/250,000 population 1 basic emergency obstetric care facility/ 125,000 population 1 comprehensive emergency obstetric care facility/500,000 population 10 hospital beds/10,000 population

Ratio of health workforce/population:
  clinician (e.g. doctor, nurse, midwife)
  community health worker
	22/10,000 population
	10/10,000

Proportion of health workforce female	50%
Outpatient consultation rate	1–4 new visits per person per year
Consultations per clinician per day	< 50
Births assisted by skilled attendant	90%
Expected deliveries by caesarean section	≥ 5% and ≥ 15%
Health facilities using universal precautions	100%
Blood for transfusion screened for transfusion-transmissible infections, including HIV	100%

Source: Sphere (2011); Pavignani and Colombo (2009: Module 12).

Note should be made of interruption to pre-existing programmes (e.g. tuberculosis, mental health, HIV, and opiate substitution therapies) and the magnitude of the disruption, including the number of people affected, likely complications and relevant consequences.

Health information system

A coordinated health information system, using standardized reporting formats, regular health service reporting, and prompt routine data analysis, reporting, and feedback, is important to ensure that services are oriented towards the most important causes of consultation and to promptly identify changing trends. Data should usually include (Sphere, 2011):

- deaths recorded by health facilities, including deaths of children under age 5
- proportional mortality
- cause-specific mortality
- incidence rates for common morbidities
- proportional morbidity
- health facility usage rate
- number of consultations per clinician per day

The existence of a functioning disease early warning system (e.g. **EWARN**) can detect suspected outbreaks early to enable rapid assessment and response and prevent avoidable morbidity and mortality. The primary purpose of an early warning system is prompt detection of outbreaks (see Chapter 8).

Health workforce

Assessments usually include an overview of working health staff, whether health staff left as a result of the crisis, and investigation of health staff capacity within displaced populations. Assessments should determine whether health staff are receiving a regular salary and any likelihood of disruption to salary systems. Initial assessments may identify information gaps in health workforce capacity and training needs for in-depth assessment.

Medical supplies and equipment

Assessment should include availability of medical supplies and equipment and functioning cold chain. Information needs include identification of specific gaps in medicines and equipment and assessment of the medicine supply chain (e.g. storage, transport, supply systems) to identify risks of future disruption. Initial assessment may identify data needs for follow-up in subsequent assessment.

Leadership and governance

Existing coordination mechanisms, strengths and weaknesses should be assessed briefly. The presence and credibility of the ministry of health or lead health agency should be noted. Observations should be noted on functioning of coordination mechanisms, proportion of actors participating regularly, degree of information provision, active harmonization of activities, identification of gaps and overlaps, and planning for future activities.

Health financing

In emergencies, health care should be available free of charge (Sphere, 2011). Initial assessment should attempt to determine whether people are required to pay for consultations or medicines and to what degree this prevents people accessing services. Detailed central-level assessment will later examine the capacity of the ministry of health and donors to pay for salaries, medicines and other routine costs following the crisis.

Activity 6.2

Using the Côte d'Ivoire case study, identify the key assessment information required now that your organization has access to the West of the country and is considering establishing health programmes there.

Data collection methods and interpretation

Assessment data can be quantitative (e.g. community surveys) or qualitative (e.g. focus groups, individual interviews). Sources can be primary (i.e. collected by the assessment team) or secondary (i.e. using existing data, such as published literature, agency reports, and health records).

Primary quantitative data

Survey data are collected by household (e.g. access to water and sanitation) or from individual household members (e.g. nutritional status). Surveys can collect data on more than one outcome of interest (e.g. vaccination coverage, food, water, nutritional status, health status). *Population surveys* aim to collect information from the whole affected population, either through *exhaustive methods* (i.e. whole population) where the population is small or *representative methods*, a quicker approach that uses fewer resources.

Several representative methods are used, including systematic and random sampling. *Systematic sampling* selects a sample population at regular intervals from the total population (e.g. if the affected population is organized in an ordered camp, every fifth house might be selected). *Random sampling* ensures every person has the same chance of being selected. A *simple random sample* may be selected by selecting five people at random from a numbered list of 100 people. For health and nutrition assessments, two-stage *cluster sampling* is often used (e.g. 30 clusters of 30 children are selected from a population). Survey results are usually presented with 95% confidence intervals, meaning the true prevalence will fall within these confidence intervals 95% of the time if the survey is conducted repeatedly. Only those with adequate expertise should conduct surveys. Technical and communication skills are required, particularly where findings may be politically sensitive (Médecins Sans Frontières, 2006).

Population size and demographic breakdown

Estimation methods include the following:

- *Systematic registration* (e.g. everyone attending food distribution, new arrivals) or, in stable situations with adequate time and resources, conducting a population census.

- *Exhaustive enumeration* (i.e. counting) of every household, often possible in small populations using direct observation or aerial photographs. Random household sampling can estimate the average number of persons per household. The two figures are multiplied to estimate total population.
- *Aerial sampling* can provide a population estimate by multiplying total area (in square metres) by population density. Density, or number of inhabitants per square metre, is estimated from a random sample taken among the affected population.

Mortality

Rates of mortality can be estimated by *counting graves*.

Retrospective mortality surveys are conducted verbally with a representative sample of households, and can collect data on cause of death, although such information is often unreliable (a more detailed diagnosis of causes of death uses *verbal autopsy* methods, but requires time, resources and skills not typically available during the initial phase of a humanitarian response). These surveys can be subject to a number of biases, including recall bias (incorrect memory).

Some form of *surveillance system* should be used to collect prospective mortality data.

Morbidity

Data are usually available through prospective data collection from health facilities, with proportional morbidity more readily available in emergencies. Calculating incidence rates requires some knowledge of the size of the population to which data refer and consistency of reporting from health facilities (e.g. if data are gathered from several facilities but not all report regularly, disease fluctuations may occur due to reporting rates rather than disease incidence in the community).

Malnutrition

Wasting, a marker of acute malnutrition is presented as a weight-for-height index, and usually measured through **anthropometric** surveys of children aged 6–59 months, for whom international weight and height reference tables exist with which to compare results. Information on context (e.g. causes of morbidity and mortality, seasonality) and underlying causes of malnutrition (e.g. food insecurity, care practices, health environment) should be considered before conducting a survey. Conducting anthropometric surveys requires specific skills and findings must be interpreted in context. Results are usually presented as percentage of the median and Z-scores (a statistical reference) as compared to reference weight and height tables.

Needs data

Recent guidance for ranking needs from a representative sample of the population has been developed using the Humanitarian Emergency Settings Perceived Needs Scale (HESPER). This asks members of affected populations to rank areas of importance to them and includes questions in 26 domains, listed in Table 6.5 (WHO, 2011a).

Table 6.5 Humanitarian Emergency Settings Perceived Needs Scale (HESPER) question domains

1. Drinking water
2. Food
3. Place to live in
4. Toilets
5. Keeping clean
6. Clothes, shoes, bedding or blankets
7. Income or livelihood
8. Physical health
9. Health care
10. Distress
11. Safety
12. Education for your children
13. Care for family members
14. Support from others
15. Separation from family members
16. Being displaced from home
17. Information
18. The way aid is provided
19. Respect
20. Moving between places
21. Too much free time
22. Law and justice in your community
23. Safety or protection from violence for women in your community
24. Alcohol or drug use in your community
25. Mental illness in your community
26. Care for people in your community who are on their own

Source: WHO (2011a).

Primary qualitative data

Community assessment enables systematic collection and analysis of primary data. Alongside the HESPER, which uses a *probability sample* of the population, additional qualitative information is collected to help organizations account for needs and priorities perceived by affected populations.

Key informant interviews gather information on community beliefs and practices from those with first-hand knowledge of the affected population (e.g. health workers, community leaders). Usually non-probabilistic sampling is used to achieve cultural representation through a range of respondents. Interviews can be *structured*, using a standard questionnaire, or in-depth (semi-structured or unstructured), using a topic guide and open-ended questions to allow probing on relevant topics.

Focus group discussions obtain collective information about perceptions and practices through interactive discussion between group members. They require considerable skill for effective facilitation and analysis.

Observation allows analysis of social behaviour as it happens, in the context in which it occurs, through watching and listening (e.g. how people wash their hands, how health staff speak to patients).

Intervention mapping – who is doing what, when, and where (known as the 'four Ws') – can give a comprehensive overview of all actors working in each sector, what activities are taking place in which locations, and planned start and end times.

Health facility assessment is likely to include structured inventory of services provided, staff present, equipment and medicines available, storage facilities, quality of medical records and possibly quality of consultation. This may follow initial assessment.

Secondary data sources

Collation and analysis of secondary information can assist in priority setting, particularly in early stages of crises if this information is readily available, as time for gathering primary data is limited. For example, context can initially be explored through literature review (e.g. published articles and grey literature, such as agency documents, websites and blogs), in addition to community consultation. Secondary sources include pre- and post-crisis information and can be qualitative and quantitative. An online search of relevant global websites – e.g. ReliefWeb (http://reliefweb.int/countries), Demographic and Health Surveys (http://www.measuredhs.com) – can be a useful starting point.

As population size estimation may be challenging, particularly in urban and diffuse settings, population data can sometimes be collected through available food distribution or refugee registration lists or extrapolated from programme data (e.g. measles vaccination, water usage data). Data from different sources should be compared and reviewed for possible biases and inaccuracies.

Crisis magnitude and severity

First, an attempt should be made to judge the magnitude and severity of the crisis. Magnitude is usually assessed as the number of people affected or at risk. Crude mortality rate (CMR), **under-5 mortality rate** (U5MR), and nutritional status of children under 5 can be used to assess the severity of an emergency. In major crises, mortality rates and malnutrition may be elevated. Table 6.6 provides alert thresholds for severe emergencies. These are presented as a rough guide, as severity needs to be interpreted in context with other elements taken into account (e.g. political and food security, population health status).

Table 6.6 Assessing the severity of an acute humanitarian crisis

Interpretation	CMR (deaths/10,000/day)	U5MR (deaths/10,000/day)	GAM* prevalence among children 6–59 months
Out of control	**> 2**	**> 4**	–
Very serious	**1–2**	**2–4**	**20%**
Alert	*> 1.0*	*> 2*	*10–19%*
Under control	< 1.0	< 2	<10%
Baseline, sub-Saharan Africa	0.5	1	5%

Source: Darcy and Hofman (2003).

* GAM is global acute malnutrition and defined as a Z-score below −2 or less than 80% median weight-for-height when compared with international reference tables.

U5MR is considered a more sensitive indicator of magnitude than CMR. A doubling of baseline mortality, a CMR higher than 1 per 10,000 population per day, or a U5MR higher than 2 per 10,000 per day indicates a major public health emergency requiring immediate intervention. As mortality information can be difficult to obtain in crises and can be politically sensitive, other severity indicators may be required, particularly in low-mortality or prolonged crises.

Acute malnutrition (wasting) among children aged 6–59 months is considered a sensitive indicator of crisis magnitude. A number of frameworks for interpretation exist, as use of absolute thresholds may be misleading. Data must be interpreted in context, including examination of trends, seasonality, food security, and overall public health.

Sharing assessment information

Assessment findings should be shared with affected populations, other partners, and health authorities. This can be through the clusters or other sectoral system activated in-country and through websites such as ReliefWeb (http://reliefweb.int) and OneResponse (http://oneresponse.info). Often systems for centralization, collation, analysis and access of assessment information will be established in affected countries.

Prioritizing responses

Various pieces of assessment information will inform intervention prioritization.

- *Principal causes of avoidable mortality, morbidity and disability* depend on the type of crisis and change over time due to environmental risk factors, increasing malnutrition, change in behavioural practices and decreased access to health services (e.g. following an acute crisis, a likely principal cause in the first week will be trauma, while morbidity and mortality from water-borne and **vector-borne diseases** and acute respiratory infections are likely to increase and become principal causes from the second week onwards). The main causes of mortality and morbidity will depend on the main endemic health problems and details of the crisis (e.g. if displaced, both in areas of origin pre-crisis and in host areas).
- *Main foreseeable health risks* may be predicted from pre-crisis health information and type of crisis (e.g. water-borne diseases are likely to increase due to flooding and in camps with inadequate access to water, sanitation and hygiene facilities; measles outbreaks are more likely in densely-populated areas with low measles immunization coverage). Importantly, if measles vaccination coverage is below 90% or unknown, mass measles vaccination campaigns for children aged 6 months to 15 years are indicated, accompanied by administration of vitamin A to children aged 6–59 months. Campaigns should cover at least 95% of target populations.
- *Vulnerable populations* should be identified, and may include unaccompanied minors, women-headed households, elderly, and people living with disability or HIV, depending on context.
- *Contextual factors* affecting health status, health services and possible humanitarian health action could include climate, topography, geography, humanitarian access and security, and cultural, economic, and sociostructural issues. These may already be identified from initial rapid assessments and do not need repeating in health assessments. Health problems will vary within a country, which may not be reflected in

national health data. Climate has significant impact on disease, while topography, humanitarian access and security can constrain the type and scale of response.

- *Capacity* available to respond includes all resources required to respond to the specific crisis (e.g. human resources, equipment, medicines, logistics, finances). This includes government, community, local and international organizational resources, and the speed with which these can be mobilized.
- *Critical gaps in geographic or sectoral coverage* are usually identified with a four Ws intervention matrix.
- *Community priorities* and participation of affected communities is recognized as essential to humanitarian response.
- *Cost-effectiveness of interventions and resource requirements* are considered when setting priorities, as finite resources can be mobilized for any responses.

Prioritization involves deciding which sectors, and which interventions within them, are most likely to have the greatest impact on most people in affected populations (e.g. in the health sector after an earthquake, trauma response may be prioritized for the first two weeks, followed by ensuring access to primary health care, reproductive health services, immunization campaigns, and health promotion interventions). Activities must include all those in need, while taking incremental steps to ensure population self-sufficiency. The prioritization process should incorporate planning for how interventions will change with time and the changing health situation, context and focus (e.g. increasing focus on recovery). Initial assessment should result in specific recommendations for initial health response activities, how these activities should change over time, and what detailed follow-up assessments are required.

Activity 6.3

In the Côte d'Ivoire case study, how could assessment information be obtained?

Conclusions

Initial assessment is a structured approach to identifying humanitarian needs and response priorities. Assessment methods and approaches vary according to agency needs, the specific context and magnitude of the humanitarian crisis, and the timing of the assessment. Common to all approaches is description of magnitude and severity of the crisis, identification of important causes and risks to population mortality, morbidity and suffering, and response capacities and gaps. Assessment findings are used to identify priority interventions, thus helping provide the greatest impact for affected populations. The next chapter will cover health service delivery priorities.

Feedback on Activities

Feedback on Activity 6.1

Your recommendation will depend on what else you can find out about the context, including how many other agencies also obtained access or are willing to provide technical and financial support. Ideally, you might recommend a multi-sectoral rapid assessment if this is feasible. However, an individual agency assessment may be the most realistic option.

Feedback on Activity 6.2

Your list may be longer, but should at least include the following essential information:

- Estimation of the magnitude and severity of the crisis: data on the size of the affected population, including movements in and out of the affected area and absorption limits of host villages, and mortality and malnutrition rates if available.
- Main causes of avoidable mortality, morbidity and disability, including any recent rumours or reports of outbreaks.
- Main foreseeable health risks (including infectious disease outbreaks), based on current and pre-crisis information, vaccination coverage, health service accessibility, essential needs coverage, season, climate, geography, and local vectors.
- Vulnerable populations, which might include female or child-headed households, people living with HIV.
- Other contextual factors: political, protection, and human rights situations.
- Capacity assessment: existing resources among governmental, national and international actors, which should include a brief analysis of the health system pre-crisis and likely impact of the crisis.
- Priority needs identified by the community.
- Critical gaps in coverage of health and other services.
- Resources and costs required to fill critical gaps and meet priority needs.
- Gaps in key information and areas requiring further in-depth or sub-sectoral assessment.

Feedback on Activity 6.3

An initial rapid assessment is indicated as very little up-to-date assessment information is available. This assessment should be multi-sectoral if at all possible, as there are indications of problems across many sectors relevant to population health (e.g. shelter, water, sanitation and hygiene, food, health). Ideally, information will be obtained through an initial multi-sectoral rapid assessment, collecting a mix of primary and secondary data to describe the overall impact of the crisis and identify priority needs and key responses. Secondary data could be collected from functioning health services, locally available documents, and published reports or other literature. Primary data could be collected through interviews and surveys. The team should aim to harmonize assessment information with that obtained from other organizations (e.g. by using common indicators) and share findings with regional and national coordination mechanisms for collation and analysis of all assessment reports.

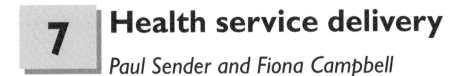

7 | Health service delivery

Paul Sender and Fiona Campbell

Overview

The aim of this chapter is to describe delivery of health services in conflict-affected settings. Concepts from programme management and humanitarian literature are used to consider who needs services, what options exist for ensuring access, how services can best be delivered by a range of actors, and links between service delivery, equity and wider system performance.

Learning outcomes

After completing this chapter you should be able to:

- describe health service delivery, including aims and challenges during conflict
- identify service delivery approaches, mechanisms and roles of different actors
- consider the role of health service delivery in supporting the humanitarian principles, health system strengthening and equity in conflict-affected settings

What is health service delivery?

Definition

The World Health Organization defines **health service delivery** as the 'provision of the promotive, preventive and curative services required to ensure health within the population'. This can be conceptualized as the relationship between policy-makers, service providers, and service consumers, and encompasses both services and supporting systems (Slaymaker and Christiansen, 2005).

Aims

The aims of health services are to deliver health care that is effective, safe and of acceptable quality, all vital components of the *right to health*. The aim of health service delivery in conflict-affected settings is to ensure people's right to health and to receive humanitarian assistance. While these rights are underpinned by international law (see Chapter 5), conflict affects health service provision and thus realization of this right – both in terms of increased needs and the ability of health systems to respond. Health needs are often acute, while access to conflict-affected populations is worsened and infrastructure and delivery capacity often disrupted. Objectives in conflict-affected settings are often narrowed to delivery of basic services to meet essential needs (e.g. primary health care, emergency surgery).

Health challenges of conflict

Conflict generates additional health needs and affects vulnerable groups both directly and indirectly (see Chapter 3). Some diseases may increase due to favourable conditions (e.g. overcrowding, unsafe water supplies), while others may be exacerbated through disruption of routine health services (e.g. immunization); see Checchi et al. (2007). Four major infectious causes (respiratory infections, diarrhoea, measles, and malaria where endemic) account for 60–90% of deaths among conflict-affected populations, often exacerbated by malnutrition.

Chronic diseases (e.g. coronary heart disease, hypertension, diabetes, respiratory diseases) can worsen in emergencies, becoming major health issues among older people. Those with chronic diseases requiring long-term management (e.g. HIV, tuberculosis) may be at increased risk due to treatment disruptions, with added potential for promoting drug resistance. Mental health is often a major concern. Sexual violence is an increasingly visible issue in conflict, affecting predominately women and girls. Sexual violence may be used strategically for military purposes, with severe psychological and physical health implications, including risk of HIV infection. These issues, combined with health burden prior to conflict, influence service provision in conflict-affected settings.

Challenges to health service delivery in conflict

While health needs often increase, ability to deliver health services may be severely constrained. Effective health service delivery depends on several key factors, including the capabilities of the health system prior to conflict and resource availability (e.g. trained and motivated staff, essential equipment and drugs, information to make informed decisions, and finances to keep the system running); see WHO (2012). Access and security may be particularly difficult in conflict settings, and negotiations across a range of actors may be required for health activities to take place. Approaches to accessing affected populations include **negotiated access** and working with community actors (Glaser, 2003).

Conflict can reduce and disrupt resources to the health system. In some countries, government public services may already be limited due to long-term under-investment and further undermined by conflict. Infrastructure is often destroyed and equipment and drugs damaged or stolen. Staff may have left their posts, be restricted in their movements due to insecurity, or even directly targeted by violence (ICRC, 2011). For example, in Liberia the pre-war number of 237 doctors was reduced to 20 at the time of the peace agreement (Interagency Health Evaluation, 2005). Health service financing may be severely disrupted during conflict, leaving staff with irregular or no salaries and unable to maintain even basic health services. Health system coping strategies may thus include introduction of formal or informal user fees, negatively impacting population access. Large influxes of displaced populations may overwhelm the capacity of already weakened health systems, undermining the quality of care and potentially increasing tensions between host and displaced populations.

Traditionally, conflict was associated with large refugee populations in camp settings. Contemporary intra-state armed conflicts are increasingly characterized by internally displaced populations and dispersed settlements (Golaz, 2010). While this may be less a reflection of choices than of available opportunities (e.g. neighbouring countries may be unwilling to open borders), the shift to internal dispersed settlements and middle-income countries affects the nature of health service delivery (Spiegel et al., 2010a).

The programmatic distinction between conflict and post-conflict can be unclear in practice.

Activity 7.1

Consider a current conflict with which you are somewhat familiar. What factors influence health service delivery? Who are the main health service delivery actors? What seems unique about the conflict you have chosen and how might this affect health service delivery?

Health service delivery roles and approaches

Role of the humanitarian community

While ensuring access to health services is the responsibility of governing authorities, both formal and de facto, where services are inadequate or authorities are unwilling to ensure their provision, the role of international humanitarian agencies is often critical. International non-governmental organizations (INGOs) are major providers of health services in conflict-affected countries. In an example from Liberia, an estimated 70% of the health facilities (i.e. approximately 200 clinics) were supported by INGOs and other agencies (Interagency Health Evaluation, 2005).

Coordination of actors and efforts

The wide range of actors supporting the delivery of health services in conflict, together with their differing remits and aims, means they are often working in an uncoordinated and sometimes contradictory manner. The coordination of efforts is therefore vital to ensure the most effective and efficient delivery of services, especially considering access and resource constraints. A range of coordination structures, such as the cluster approach, may be in place to support coordination. However, while organizations may be generally supportive of the principle of coordination, disagreements over the mechanisms used and challenges reconciling coordination with agency remits are common.

Health service delivery approaches and mechanisms

Agencies may adopt one or more positions in their support for health service delivery, working within the national system or in parallel, though the latter is rarer. Context, agency remit, phase of the emergency, and health system capacity will determine the approach or approaches adopted. Service delivery approaches may place a greater or lesser emphasis on health system support.

Agencies that prioritize working with national systems may support existing health staff and structures to function more effectively through provision of drugs and equipment, salary support and staff supervision. Health services are delivered in accordance with national policies and plans, although agencies may advocate that these be adapted to ensure service quality. This approach, while providing opportunity to support and strengthen existing systems during conflict, may present challenges to quality and reach.

Agencies that prioritize immediate life-saving care generally invest heavily in placing their own staff within existing health structures, providing intensive logistical and budgetary support, and international procurement of drugs and equipment. This approach can mean higher quality and sometimes greater reach. However, these investments are less sustainable than strengthening existing capacity and in some cases can even undermine the existing system, leaving it no better and sometimes in a poorer condition once the acute crisis is over.

Delivery mechanisms can include parallel, mobile, community-based, public–private and military delivery.

Though less common, agencies may choose to work in parallel with existing health services, providing direct care through their own facilities and staff. This may occur where there is no pre-existing national health system or when government is unwilling to work in partnership, but willing to provide access. The benefits of this delivery method include the potential to provide high-quality care, but options for sustainability or longer-term support to the system are limited. Health care provision in camp settings is usually parallel. Due to the absence of pre-existing health facilities and the temporary nature of camps, ambitions for sustainability are generally not applicable.

Mobile delivery may be used in some cases, including as parallel service provision, to provide useful access to hard-to-reach or mobile populations with little or no access to fixed facilities. Mobile units can provide a selected range of health services and a referral system. However, they are controversial due to the cost and intermittent nature of the services they provide. Ideally, they should be used exceptionally where there is no alternative for accessing the health system (du Mortier and Coninx, 2007).

Humanitarian agencies may also work with or through national civil society groups, potentially extending their reach to areas inaccessible to international agencies (e.g. areas affected by conflict). Community-based approaches can also contribute to broader service delivery objectives and may be vital in conflict and emergency situations (GHWA et al., 2011). Health services supported at community level include a wide range of interventions such as health promotion and some curative services. Their potential is maximized when linkages with trained health staff and fixed health facilities are strengthened (Lehmann and Sanders, 2007).

A domestic private sector may flourish in the absence of a functioning public health system and international private practitioners may enter the health care system when opportunities present, as has occurred in Iraq and Afghanistan. While opportunities for delivery partnerships exist, humanitarian health actors may find it challenging to work alongside the private sector, particularly if motives do not align.

In some contexts the military – both national and international – may be involved in delivery of health services. This increasing trend reflects responsibilities as de facto authorities in situations of occupation and an increase in the **hearts and minds agenda** as part of wider political objectives. The increase of military health service delivery alongside humanitarian delivery is causing concern within the humanitarian community, both for the safety of humanitarian staff, who may be confused with military targets, and reduced access to populations receiving military health services.

Addressing essential health needs

Health services address population health needs by restoring and maintaining health. However, providing comprehensive health services in conflict-affected environments is very difficult. Thus, prioritizing **essential health services** is necessary. Defining what is essential depends on the particular conflict. However, essential services should address the main health problems within a population and prevent and reduce excess mortality and morbidity (Sphere, 2011). Due to the high disease burden of infectious diseases, these should be included in any essential services package. Additionally, child health, sexual and reproductive health, and mental health services are needed. Injury and trauma services are likely to be needed depending on the course of the conflict (Sphere, 2011). Non-communicable diseases may be prevalent, particularly in populations with a large proportion of older people, and should be considered as part of an essential package.

Essential service packages

Difficult decisions are often required in developing an essential service package, as resources and capacity are often constrained. A range of minimum packages exist to address specific health issues and support service delivery decisions. Examples include the **Minimum Initial Service Package** (MISP) for reproductive health, designed to address the most important causes of reproductive morbidity and mortality among women, men and adolescents in the acute phase of disasters and conflict (RHRC, 2011). Other agencies have designed their own intervention packages, which can be tailored to the specific context.

Activity 7.2

The MISP self-study module is currently available at http://misp.rhrc.org/. If possible, go online and review the module. What services does the MISP cover? Do you think additional services should be included?

As health and service needs change over time, the initial essential package will need to be expanded to address an increasingly comprehensive range of health issues as circumstances permit. For example, the MISP is designed to be expanded when circumstances allow, while UNICEF's emergency health and nutrition interventions are categorized in two phases – the first lasting 6–8 weeks and the second for the period after the initial response (UNICEF, 2012).

Service packages designed and implemented during conflict may provide valuable lessons for scale-up of services in the post-conflict period. NGO primary health care services, implemented during extended conflict in Afghanistan, were developed into a national basic package of health services (BPHS) by the Ministry of Public Health following the war. As a general guide, Overseas Development Institute (ODI) criteria for selecting optimal services suggest interventions should:

- address the main health problems in a population
- be feasible in terms of implementation
- have the potential to maximize benefits
- maximize effectiveness and be the best cost for the outcome
- be timely in terms of preventing outbreaks or an increased health burden

The wider role of health service delivery

Humanitarian principles in health service delivery

For health service delivery to be effective, populations must be able to access services when required. The concept that access should be on the basis of need is supported by international humanitarian law. The humanitarian principles of humanity, independence, impartiality, and neutrality thus provide a framework for delivery of humanitarian assistance, including health service delivery (see Chapter 5). Not all health service actors view the humanitarian principles as relevant to their actions. For example, governmental and non-governmental military actors may have strategic purposes, not related to need, for supporting health service delivery.

For humanitarian agencies, these principles are essential in negotiating access to target populations, particularly demonstrating impartiality (or for some agencies neutrality) and independence. Thus, ensuring service delivery decision-making is aligned with humanitarian principles is crucial for humanitarian agencies such as ICRC. This can involve assessing all actions for their impact on independence, impartiality and neutrality and working to support service delivery according to all three. This may be challenging, and compromises are often required in the negotiation process.

The involvement of government funding in humanitarian health service delivery can represent a compromise of humanitarian principles, if the government in question is overly politically or militarily involved in the country concerned. In some cases, agencies resolve this by declining government funds for their work in countries in which that government is involved (e.g. some health agencies declined funding from USAID during the second Gulf War). Some agencies, such as Médecins Sans Frontières, have built up significant private income – seeing financial independence as pivotal to working according to their principles and delivering health care according to needs alone. Financial independence may provide additional service delivery options when balancing the ability to act quickly with use of available assets, particularly if these are government or military assets. Independence can also allow for health service delivery in areas that do not match donor priorities. However, receipt of institutional funding (i.e. from government donors) does not necessarily lead to a lack of independence, as the ICRC's role and mandate illustrate. The increasing politicization of humanitarian aid has left many humanitarian agencies fearful of the impact on humanitarian principles and action (Egeland et al., 2011).

Activity 7.3

During the Angolan conflict, agencies provided equivalent health care in both government-held and UNITA-held areas, ensuring cooperation of both sides and thus neutrality. While this may have been a neutral act, it was not necessarily an impartial one if needs had been greater in UNITA-held than in government-held areas. How would you ensure neutrality is preserved in delivery of health services in a conflict-affected setting?

Links between health service delivery and longer-term health system strengthening

The aim of **health system strengthening** is to ensure access to quality health care that addresses population needs. It requires supporting efforts by the ministry of health, national stakeholders, and communities, to take ownership of the health system. This may require capacity development of local actors to ensure they are able to run the health system effectively. The service delivery contributions of external NGOs and other agencies may be significant, though this is often a reflection on the poor state of the existing health system. However, all engagement in health service delivery presents an opportunity to ensure that the health system is not undermined.

Accountability within health service delivery is critical and can be viewed from a number of angles. Not only do agencies working to support health service delivery need to be accountable to the populations that use the services and any funders supporting their efforts, accountability must also focus on the responsibility of the state to its citizens. Supporting state responsibility is part of any programme to strengthen the health system. Health system strengthening is covered in more detail in Chapter 13.

Promoting equity of access to health services in conflict

Conflict and state fragility are critical drivers of health inequity. In DRC, research indicated that conflict-affected areas had 2–3 times higher morbidity and mortality than non-conflict-affected areas (Bornemisza et al., 2010). Displacement, gender issues, access to markets and food security are all significant contributing factors to inequities in health status, in turn exacerbated by inequality of health service access. The way health services are planned and delivered may affect this significantly. For example, the use of financing approaches that restrict access to services, such as user fees, may be a major factor in inequity.

A number of challenges arise for promoting equity in health service delivery in conflict-affected settings. In some contexts, health care provided within camps has been of a higher standard than that provided to resident populations outside camps (Spiegel et al., 2010a). Although the original intention was to address inequalities in morbidity and mortality, high-quality parallel health services can ultimately create disparities in the opposite direction. Agencies attempting to address this will rarely provide support to populations within a camp without promoting access to those outside. However, host populations may perceive that those in camps receive better services, even if this is not the case.

Support to one part of the system and not another, while addressing access for some, may create inequity within the overall health system. In Liberia, NGO support to health facilities was focused on the areas worst hit by the war and was not evenly spread throughout the country (Interagency Health Evaluation, 2005). While these areas were considered most in need, no agency had oversight of what this meant for health services in the country as a whole. For some agencies, therefore, avoidance of inequity rather than promotion of equity is the major driving concern. Identifying ways to address health needs without promoting inequity then determines the approach to health service delivery.

There are no simple solutions to the delivery of equitable health services in conflict situations, but understanding where services are currently being provided and who is accessing them is vital in determining the impact on equity and thus choosing solutions. As conflict is the key social determinant of health in these contexts, addressing health inequalities in conflict-affected contexts is ultimately about addressing conflict itself.

Conclusions

Health service delivery in conflict-affected settings aims to ensure people's right to health and to receive humanitarian assistance. However, conflict presents particular challenges for those attempting to deliver services, whether as public providers or humanitarian community actors. Designing programmes to address needs, while ensuring equity and support to longer-term health system strengthening, is a continuing challenge. Recent humanitarian responses across a range of conflict-affected countries have demonstrated the need to consider context-specific issues, including the ability of the health system to respond. The next chapter discusses infectious disease control in conflict-affected settings.

Feedback on activities

Feedback on Activity 7.1

Your answer will reflect the conflict you have chosen. However, some factors you have probably considered include disease burden, health needs, population dynamics, and the state of the current health system. Health delivery actors normally include national and international actors, though this depends on both interest and access for the latter. Context is paramount. You may have chosen a forgotten conflict that has not attracted the attention of the international community, in which case those delivering services will be predominately national health staff. Additionally, services may only be available in localized areas as staff cannot travel. Alternatively, you may have chosen a high-profile conflict, with a large international presence and many actors involved in service delivery.

Feedback on Activity 7.2

MISP recommends a coordinated set of priority activities, for implementation in the early days and weeks of an emergency, designed to prevent and manage the consequences of sexual violence, prevent excess neonatal and maternal morbidity and mortality, reduce HIV transmission, and plan for comprehensive reproductive health services. You may argue that other services, such as HIV treatment, should be provided.

Feedback on Activity 7.3

As neutrality can be both perceived and actual, it is important that others see you and your agency as neutral. You may wish to examine how health services are delivered, including who is delivering and receiving them, to be sure there is no possibility of suggesting your agency is taking sides. You would probably want to ensure that you are basing your responses on health need and that you look for ways to address health needs that do not promote or favour one party over the other. Additionally, consider whether your efforts to appear neutral could be jeopardizing your impartiality.

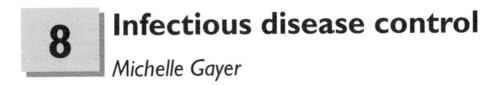

8 Infectious disease control

Michelle Gayer

Overview

The aim of this chapter is to provide an overview of infectious disease control in conflict-affected humanitarian emergencies, focusing on priority infectious diseases. Concepts from epidemiological research and disease control in humanitarian emergencies are used to describe control priorities.

Learning outcomes

After completing this chapter you should be able to:

- identify risk factors for infectious disease transmission during conflict, including which infectious diseases cause the greatest burden of morbidity and mortality
- conduct an infectious disease risk assessment in a conflict-affected setting
- describe key interventions for infectious disease control during conflict, including principles of surveillance and epidemic response

Conflict and infectious diseases

Humanitarian emergencies caused by conflict are frequently characterized by the displacement of large numbers of people. Those affected are often resettled in temporary locations with high population densities, inadequate food and shelter, unsafe water and poor sanitation. These conditions enable infectious diseases, either alone or in combination with malnutrition, to emerge as major causes of morbidity and mortality. Multiple risk factors may interact to produce higher incidences of diarrhoeal diseases, acute respiratory infections (ARI), vaccine-preventable diseases (e.g. measles), and vector-borne diseases (e.g. malaria). Tuberculosis and HIV are also major health concerns that can be amplified by these conditions. In such contexts, surveillance for early detection of and response to epidemics and infectious disease prevention and control interventions are critical to reducing excess morbidity and mortality.

Risk factors increasing infectious disease transmission

Numerous risk factors for transmission of infectious diseases may be exacerbated by conflict. To prevent and control infectious diseases, and therefore reduce excess morbidity and mortality, it is imperative to understand the key risk factors that increase infectious disease transmission in conflict. Note that the risk factors for infectious disease transmission do not inherently change but can be enhanced by conflict. These can be categorized into the classical *host–agent–environment* **epidemiological triad**.

Host factors

High malnutrition levels. Under-nutrition or malnutrition may develop over prolonged periods of conflict and food scarcity. Malnutrition compromises natural immunity, leading to increased susceptibility to infection and more frequent and severe episodes of infectious diseases. Likewise, infection can aggravate or precipitate malnutrition through decreased appetite and intake, malabsorption, nutrient loss or increased metabolic needs. Finally, severe malnutrition often masks symptoms and signs of infectious diseases, making prompt clinical diagnosis and early treatment difficult. The synergistic combination of malnutrition and infectious diseases is a major public health problem, particularly among infants and children. Among young children, mortality is associated with malnutrition in over 60% of deaths resulting from diarrhoea, over 50% of deaths as a result of pneumonia and malaria, and over 40% of deaths as a result of measles. Under-nutrition and micronutrient deficiencies can also increase the morbidity and mortality from infectious diseases (Caulfield et al., 2004).

Low immunization coverage levels. This may occur due to disruptions in routine vaccination programmes with prolonged conflict but also due to spoiling of vaccines if appropriate **cold chain** temperature and transport conditions are not maintained. Vaccine-preventable diseases important in conflict include respiratory droplet spread infections (i.e. measles, pertussis, diphtheria, meningococcal meningitis), polio (spread faecal-orally), and tetanus (acquired through contaminated wounds, although not transmissible from human to human).

Community cultural practices and behaviours. Consumption of bush meat or close proximity to domestic animals, unsafe sexual practices or intravenous drug use, and some funeral practices may promote transmission of infectious diseases. Certain behaviours may intensify with conflict (e.g. mass displacement and overcrowding may increase proximity to animals). It is vital to be aware of current practices, such as bednet usage or water boiling among communities, when planning interventions.

Relatively low immunity levels. This may promote infection in populations stressed from hunger and thirst, exhausted from having to walk long distances to flee from insecurity, having underlying chronic diseases, or simply moving from areas of low to high disease endemicity (e.g. malaria).

High concentrations of vulnerable populations. Those particularly vulnerable to infectious diseases may be concentrated among the displaced population (e.g. young children, pregnant women, elderly people).

Agent factors

Pathogen presence. A **pathogen** would usually be present in the affected area. However, it is important to consider pathogens that may be imported through displacement of populations from other areas, or from incoming international aid workers.

Disease incidence, prevalence, seasonality. Consider which **endemic** (e.g. malaria, Rift Valley fever) and **epidemic**-prone diseases (e.g. cholera, typhoid, measles, meningococcal disease) are present, their seasonality and any recent epidemics that may have occurred in recent history.

Drug resistance. Pathogens may develop resistance to anti-microbial medications, rendering these medications ineffective or sub-optimally effective against these pathogens. In conflict settings, this may occur due to inappropriate diagnosis; use of outdated and expired drugs or lack of quality control; inappropriate drug regimens; treatment disruption (e.g. due to supply chain failures, sudden displacement); and poor compliance due to purchasing inadequate quantities, selling drugs, saving drugs for future use, or health improvements after partial completion of regimen.

Disruption of infectious disease control programmes. Disruption of disease prevention and control programmes, such as routine immunization, antenatal care, and particularly vector control (e.g. insecticide spraying, larviciding, bednet distribution) may lead to significant resurgences in pathogen transmission. Malaria and other mosquito-borne (e.g. dengue, yellow fever, Japanese encephalitis, Rift Valley fever), tick-borne (e.g. Crimean–Congo haemorrhagic fever, typhus), louse-borne (e.g. epidemic typhus, relapsing fever), flea-borne (e.g. plague), or rodent-borne (e.g. leptospirosis) diseases may also be endemic in conflict-affected areas.

Environmental factors

Inadequate shelter. This increases disease risk in at least three ways. First, exposure to the elements in hot climates can lead to dehydration, especially in children, making other dehydrating diseases more severe (e.g. diarrhoea). Exposure to rain and cold temperatures favours the progression of ARI and other respiratory disease. Second, exposure to disease vectors (e.g. mosquitoes, fleas) occurs where there is inadequate roofing or walls, increasing transmission of vector-borne diseases. Furthermore, indoor residual insecticide spraying (IRS) or installing bednets is difficult in many temporary shelters. Finally, exposure to indoor smoke, due to cooking or heating inside shelters lacking proper air ventilation, is a major risk factor for ARI.

Overcrowding. This relates to *high population density* (large numbers of people per unit area), which increases contact risk between an infectious and susceptible people and thus disease transmission, and *high population concentration* (i.e. very large populations), which can result in a faster epidemic spread to many more people. For example, measles outbreaks are common, as it spreads rapidly in crowded conditions among populations with low immunization coverage. Crowded living conditions can facilitate transmission of vaccine-preventable diseases (e.g. measles, diphtheria, pertussis meningococcal meningitis), tuberculosis, diarrhoeal diseases, vector-borne diseases, and potentially increase ARI prevalence in displaced populations.

Unsafe water, inadequate sanitation and hygiene. Often the result of large-scale population displacement, these can facilitate **faecal-oral transmission** of disease. Epidemic-prone diarrhoeal diseases (e.g. cholera, typhoid fever, shigellosis) can cause high rates of mortality (e.g. Goma). Hepatitis E can result in jaundice and increased mortality in pregnant women (e.g. Darfur, Chad). Inadequate hygiene may also result in proliferation of lice, which can transmit typhus and relapsing fever.

Lack of access to health services. Health service disruptions may result from destruction, looting, flight of health staff, and ongoing conflict. The main effect of a lack of or delay in treatment is an increased case fatality rate. Longer-term programmes (e.g. those for tuberculosis, HIV and AIDS) are at significant risk from service disruptions. Rapid identification of those on treatment and prompt resumption of services are essential to ensure continuity of care. This is also crucial to reduce the risk of development and spread of drug-resistant strains such as multidrug-resistant tuberculosis and extensively drug-resistant tuberculosis. Disrupted public utilities can further lead to interruption in hospital and laboratory services; for example, if the supply of electricity is irregular then refrigeration cannot be maintained and thus drugs and vaccines cannot be stored. Difficulties in logistics and supplies may also obstruct infection control policies and practices in health care facilities, including safe blood transfusion, hand hygiene, and safe disposal of medical waste.

Poor surveillance and response systems. Weak or non-existent systems prevent early detection of outbreaks, thus delaying implementation of appropriate control measures. Detection delays combined with poor health care access, lack of effective drugs or vaccines, and lack of expertise may increase the duration of epidemics in conflict situations.

Environmental changes. If occurring in a resettlement area, these may create breeding sites (e.g. swamps, water containers, used tyres, poor drainage around shelters, lack of rubbish disposal) for vectors such as mosquitoes, flies or rodents. Population displacement from high- to low-endemicity areas, where the new environment and vector ecology are conducive to the disease, may promote new transmission of a disease that was not present before, through importation of the pathogen by the displaced population (e.g. malaria).

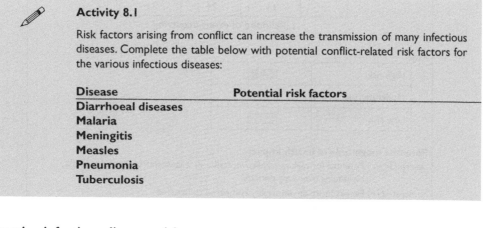

Activity 8.1

Risk factors arising from conflict can increase the transmission of many infectious diseases. Complete the table below with potential conflict-related risk factors for the various infectious diseases:

Disease	Potential risk factors
Diarrhoeal diseases	
Malaria	
Meningitis	
Measles	
Pneumonia	
Tuberculosis	

Assessing infectious diseases risk

WHO uses a modified infectious disease risk assessment process for humanitarian emergencies, adapted from methods used by other sectors. The three steps are (i) event description, (ii) threat/vulnerability assessment, and (iii) risk characterization (WHO, 2007a).

Event description is the process of systematically assessing the type of emergency and the characteristics of the displaced population. Factors such as the size of the displaced population and duration of the displacement can influence infectious disease transmission risk.

Threat/vulnerability assessment is a process that identifies potential interactions between the emergency-affected population (i.e. host), likely pathogens (i.e. agents) and exposures (i.e. environment), which determine the factors that facilitate infectious disease transmission. A comprehensive consideration of likely agents or pathogens is critical for threat assessment. Specifically, endemic and epidemic-prone diseases and their seasonality, the history of recent outbreaks and the infectious disease control programmes operating in the area must be considered. Indicators, such as those used to quantify the burden of disease or programmatic impact, are also assessed. Population factors should consider demographics, immunity, nutritional status and community practices. Environmental factors influencing infectious disease transmission, such as shelter (i.e. amount, quality, location), availability of safe water and sanitation and access to basic health care services, should also be assessed.

Risk characterization uses a risk assessment matrix to analyse the available information on hazards and exposures for each disease under consideration (Figure 8.1). Both aspects of risk – the potential magnitude of the health impact and the likelihood of the

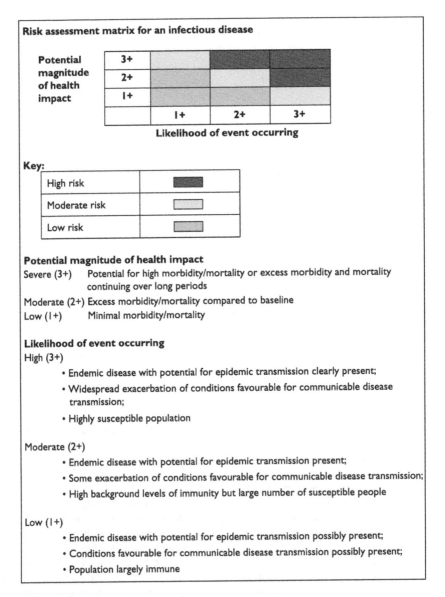

Figure 8.1 Risk characterization using a risk assessment matrix

Source: Annex 2 (WHO, 2007a).

event occurring – are quantified approximately and the overall risk is then characterized using the matrix.

Based on the overall risk assessment, disease control interventions can be prioritized by evaluating additional factors such as marginal utility, cost, availability of
resources and infrastructure requirements.

Activity 8.2

Choose the scenario described in Activity 8.3 or another conflict scenario with
which you are familiar. Consider the risk from measles, using the risk assessment
matrix provided in Figure 8.1 for your chosen area.

Key interventions for infectious disease prevention and control

Appropriately sited and sufficiently spacious shelter

Shelters must be sited with sufficient space between them, sufficient space within
them to prevent overcrowding, and adequate ventilation to prevent diseases that are
spread through respiratory droplets (e.g. measles, pneumonia, tuberculosis). Reducing
overcrowding will also help to prevent diarrhoeal and vector-borne diseases.

Safe and sufficient water, with appropriate storage

Ensuring an uninterrupted supply of safe drinking water is a critical preventive measure
in reducing the risk of water-borne diseases. WHO and the Sphere Project recommend at least 15–20 litres of safe water be provided per person per day (Sphere, 2011).
Any water source should be considered contaminated, and boiled or made safe through
treatment before it is consumed or used in food preparation. Free chlorine is the most
widely available, easily used, and affordable drinking water disinfectant option. It is
highly effective against nearly all water-borne pathogens. Provision of appropriate
water containers that can be closed or tapped will also reduce the risk of diarrhoeal
diseases and proliferation of mosquitoes.

Safe and sufficient toilet and hygiene facilities

To prevent the transmission of faecal-oral diseases, adequate sanitation and hygiene
facilities should be available in the form of latrines, or designated defecation areas, and
hand-washing facilities with soap. Latrines should be sufficient in number (i.e. one per
20 persons), sited in a safe area, be private during use, allow enough light to enter and
be well ventilated to encourage use, and be maintained regularly. Hand-washing facilities should be readily accessible upon leaving the latrine.

Safe food and appropriate cooking facilities

To ensure that the nutritional needs of the affected populations are met, access to food
of sufficient quantity and nutritional quality is important. Provision of cooking pots and

fuel, as well as education on simple measures related to food storage, preparation and consumption at household level, food handling at market level and safe water handling to avoid contamination of containers, can reduce the risk of food-borne disease. This is particularly relevant for infants, pregnant women and the elderly, who are most susceptible to food-borne diseases.

Immunization

In crowded settings, vaccination using a measles-containing vaccine, together with vitamin A supplementation, is an immediate and priority health intervention. All children aged 6 months to 15 years should receive measles vaccination, regardless of prior vaccination or disease history, with vitamin A supplementation to those aged 6–59 months. If there is ongoing poliomyelitis transmission in the area, every opportunity should be taken to give oral polio vaccine to all children under 5 years of age. When the conflict situation stabilizes, vaccinations routinely offered through the national immunization programme (e.g. measles, diphtheria, pertussis, tetanus, polio, BCG for tuberculosis, yellow fever, hepatitis B, *Haemophilus influenzae* type b, pneumococcal conjugate vaccine) should be made available to appropriate age groups as part of the essential package of health services.

Accessible primary and referral health services for case treatment

Early health care seeking and reinforcement of correct case management is important in reducing the impact of infectious diseases. The rapid diagnosis and treatment of an individual with an infectious disease reduces the duration that a person is infective and therefore prevents further disease transmission and, importantly, reduces the possibility of death. The use of symptom-based algorithms and standard treatment protocols in health facilities with agreed-upon first-line medications can ensure effective diagnosis and treatment for numerous infectious diseases. Rapid diagnostic tests, notably for malaria, should be used to prevent unnecessary treatments, although co-morbidities should also be considered in such contexts. Furthermore, infection control practices in accordance with globally accepted standard precautions should be implemented, to prevent nosocomial transmission of disease.

Epidemic surveillance and response

The primary purpose of a surveillance or early warning system during conflict is rapid detection of and response to infectious disease outbreaks. Trends in incidence of endemic diseases can also be monitored. The surveillance/early warning system should focus on the priority epidemic-prone diseases most likely to occur in the affected population. Furthermore, it should: (i) be simple, containing a small number of reportable events and including standard case definitions for the events to be used uniformly across all health facilities; (ii) include standard reporting mechanisms and forms, as well as processes for dealing with reports of potential epidemic 'alerts' from health facilities and 'rumours' from the community; (iii) complement existing surveillance structures and ensure prompt verification and investigation of alerts and rumours; (iv) identify key laboratories for confirmation of the main infectious disease threats and protocols for transport and tracking of specimens; and (v) include multi-sectoral preparedness plans for outbreak response, including pre-positioned stockpiles of drugs and supplies, identification of isolation facilities and training of health staff.

Social mobilization and risk communication

Social mobilization involves understanding people's attitudes, beliefs, and values so that communications messages are rooted in people's knowledge, understanding and perceptions of what is being recommended, obtained through trusted and credible sources (WHO, 2008b). To be effective, all disease prevention and control interventions will require compliance on the part of the community and potential behavioural change. It is therefore important to: (i) learn about current cultural and behavioural practices; (ii) identify what would motivate people to adopt desired behaviours and the most suitable way to convey the intended message, so that (iii) communication and approaches have sense and value, and promote practices that are consistent with people's cultural spheres.

Risk communication is a critical tool for outbreak control. It involves communicating about a crisis with all stakeholders – the public, government, media, other aid organizations – with the ultimate objective of controlling the outbreak (i.e. preventing further cases and minimizing death). Risk communication aims to encourage appropriate behaviours, minimize panic, and harness socioeconomic and political support for outbreak control. In whatever way messages are delivered to audiences, key principles to maintain are trust, early provision of information, transparency, and respect for public concerns. This requires careful planning, preparation, response and evaluation.

Vector control

Vectors can breed: (i) on the body (e.g. *lice*, vectors for epidemic typhus and relapsing fever); (ii) in houses (e.g. *fleas*, vectors for plague); and (iii) externally. External vector breeding can occur peridomestically in water storage (e.g. *sandflies*, vectors for cutaneous and visceral leishmaniasis; *houseflies*, vectors for amoebic dysentery, salmonellosis, hepatitis A; *aedes mosquitoes*, vectors for arboviruses including yellow fever, dengue, Rift Valley fever, West Nile fever, and Japanese encephalitis) and sewerage (e.g. *culex mosquitoes*, vectors for arboviruses and filariasis). Some vectors (e.g. many *anopheles mosquitoes*, vectors for malaria) prefer clean slow water and may breed at a greater distance from human habitation.

Integrated vector management, as promoted by WHO, requires understanding which disease-transmitting vectors are present, their biting and resting behaviours, and using available health infrastructure and resources to integrate available and effective chemical, biological or environmental measures for their control. Key vector control methods used in conflict settings are IRS of shelter walls if local vectors rest on the walls inside dwellings; insecticide-treated materials such as tents, plastic sheeting and blankets; long-lasting insecticidal nets (LLINs) that can be slept under where biting takes place after people are sleeping; larviciding of vectors that tend to breed in permanent or slow-moving water bodies; environmental management, including window screening, waste disposal, drainage, filling of swamps; and personal protection measures, such as repellents and long-sleeved or insecticide-treated clothing.

In acute emergencies, emergency shelters could initially be constructed with insecticide-treated plastic sheeting, insecticide-treated tents used, or, if shelter walls are a suitable material, IRS of all dwellings with an effective insecticide can be conducted. If rapid IRS is logistically impossible, LLINs should be distributed along with appropriate social mobilization. In areas of dengue transmission, all open water storage containers should be covered and a larvicide (e.g. Abate) added to containers that cannot be closed.

Environmental sanitation and waste disposal

Environmental sanitation and appropriate waste disposal not only contribute to vector control but also prevent contamination of water sources, promote correct use of facilities and avoid disease transmission from health facility waste. Key interventions include correct waste disposal with separation of normal waste, contaminated waste, human tissue and sharps in health facilities; incineration to decontaminate waste and avoid large refuse piles that could attract rats and flies or potentially encourage use as defecation areas; and appropriate drainage around shelters, water points, latrines and hand-washing facilities to prevent mosquitoes and flies breeding.

Activity 8.3

In March 2011, a WHO risk assessment document on Libya read as follows:

> Recent events in north Africa and the Middle East have led to unrest in a number of countries across the region. In the Libyan Arab Jamahiriya ... [mass] population movements are occurring particularly among migrant workers from [neighbouring] countries seeking repatriation. ... Estimates suggest approximately 1 million Egyptian, 80 000 Pakistani, 59 000 Sudanese, 50 000 Bangladeshi, 26 000 Filipino and 2 000 Nepalese migrant workers, as well as other nationalities from Africa and Asian migrant workers are currently employed in the Libyan Arab Jamahiriya. Despite active and coordinated repatriation efforts, the massive influx into neighbouring countries has created bottlenecks on the borders due to delays in onward transportation of workers to their home countries. Repatriation activities have now increased, but given the uncertainties surrounding the situation, it is difficult to predict the number of people that will continue to cross the border in the coming days and weeks. As of 5 March, according to estimates from Egyptian and Tunisian authorities, over 200 000 people had left the Libyan Arab Jamahiriya, crossing the borders into Egypt and Tunisia; a further 3 000 have crossed the southern border into the Niger. (WHO, 2011b)

Briefly describe the potential infectious disease risks resulting from this conflict and population displacement and categorize them according to the potential interventions that could be implemented (e.g. water-borne, vector-borne).

Conclusions

Infectious diseases can be a leading cause of morbidity and mortality in conflict situations. Violent conflicts can exacerbate existing risk factors or cause new ones (e.g. overcrowding, lack of sanitation and safe water, poor vaccination coverage, malnutrition, reduced access to appropriate treatment) that can increase pathogen transmission, progression to disease, and death. Careful assessment of context and potential host, agent and environmental risk factors, followed by risk characterization in terms of the likelihood of a disease occurring and magnitude of its potential impact, should allow considered prioritization of interventions to reduce excess morbidity and mortality. The next chapter discusses interventions for chronic diseases and broad health-related issues (e.g. disability, sexual violence).

Feedback on activities

Feedback on Activity 8.1

You could have included the following infectious disease risk factors:

Disease	Potential conflict-related risk factors
Diarrhoeal diseases	Overcrowding, inadequate amount and/or quality of water, poor personal hygiene, poor washing facilities, poor sanitation, insufficient soap, inadequate cooking facilities
Malaria	Movement from areas of low malaria endemicity to high malaria endemicity (e.g. from Rwanda to Tanzania), areas of still or slow-moving water, lack of shelter and exposure to mosquitoes, inadequate health care services, flooding
Meningitis	Meningitis belt, dry season, dust storms, overcrowding, high ARI rates
Measles	Low vaccination coverage rates, malnutrition
Pneumonia	Inadequate shelter with overcrowding and poor ventilation, indoor cooking, poor health care services, malnutrition, poor personal hygiene, age groups under 1 year old, cold weather, poor measles immunization rates
Tuberculosis	High HIV seroprevalence rates, overcrowding, malnutrition

Feedback on Activity 8.2

Your results will depend on the conflict you have chosen. Using the Libya scenario, described in Activity 8.3, you would probably conclude that while the public health impact of a measles outbreak in Libya is likely to be high (e.g. 3+), the risk was currently relatively low (e.g. 1+) due to high existing vaccination levels. For example:

Potential magnitude of health impact				
	3+	(measles Libya)		
	2+			
	1+			
		1+	**2+**	**3+**

Likelihood of event occurring

Feedback on Activity 8.3

Wounds and injuries. Given the acute conflict, wound infection and tetanus may be a problem if access to health facilities is difficult and the presentation of acute injuries is delayed. Gangrene is a complication of wound contamination, and prompt wound treatment is critical for its prevention.

WASH-related and food-borne diseases. Displaced populations and refugees arriving in Tunisia and Egypt are at potential risk from outbreaks of diseases related to reduced access to safe water, sanitation, hygiene facilities and safe food. There is a risk of typhoid fever, hepatitis A and hepatitis E. Diarrhoea is a major contributor to under-5 mortality, accounting for 8% of under-5 deaths. Cholera is not endemic in Libya.

Diseases associated with crowding. If displaced populations are housed in large (i.e. over 1,000 population), crowded transit settlements for extended periods, risk may increase of transmission of infectious diseases spread from person to person through respiratory droplets (e.g. measles, diphtheria, influenza, pertussis, meningitis, ARI – especially pneumonia). If ventilation is inadequate, this risk is increased and will include tuberculosis, an important cause of morbidity and mortality in Libya. In the acute phase of an emergency, the potential treatment interruption for all chronic diseases (e.g. tuberculosis, HIV, diabetes) and loss of patient follow-up can be a significant problem. Libya is north of the meningitis belt, so meningococcal disease is a lesser risk than in southern neighbours (e.g. Chad, Niger). Overcrowding can increase transmission of water-borne and vector-borne diseases.

Vaccine-preventable diseases. Reports from the Libyan national authorities, WHO and UNICEF in 2009 indicated high (98%) measles, diphtheria, tetanus and pertussis (DPT), and polio immunization coverage among 1-year-old children, suggesting the risk from these diseases is relatively low. However, with prolonged conflict and disruption of routine vaccination services, the pool of susceptible people will increase as children are born and not immunized.

Vector-borne disease. Literature shows little risk of vector-borne diseases. There is currently no malaria risk, although imported malaria has periodically resulted in limited local transmission and was last reported in 2003. There is currently no risk of dengue haemorrhagic fever in Libya. The risk of rabies is currently low. Scattered foci of enzootic plague exist across the country. The last outbreak of plague was reported in the Mediterranean coastal town of Tubruq in 2009, and included a cluster of five cases and one death. Population displacement in areas of known natural foci may increase the risk of exposure to rodent reservoirs of plague infection, increasing the risk of sporadic cases of plague.

Malnutrition. In 2007, the proportion of underweight children in Libya was 4.8%. If the crisis is prolonged, with a lack of access to appropriate adequate food and complementary foods, the risk of malnutrition could increase for vulnerable groups such as young children, pregnant and lactating women, and older people.

Chronic conditions and cross-cutting interventions

9

Natasha Howard, Adrianna Murphy, Rukhsana Haider, James Pallett, Jean-Francois Trani and Peter Ventevogel

Overview

The aim of this chapter is to provide an overview of chronic health care and cross-cutting health-related issues in conflict-affected areas. As conflict and the types of areas affected by conflict violence have changed, greater numbers of urban, higher-income and older populations are affected. Concepts from clinical care, public health, and epidemiology are used to describe issues and interventions relating to chronic diseases, sexual and reproductive health, nutrition, mass casualty, disability and mental health in conflict settings.

Learning outcomes

After completing this chapter you should be able to:

- explain why chronic and cross-cutting interventions are increasingly important for agencies providing health care to conflict-affected populations
- identify recommended approaches to chronic diseases, sexual and reproductive health, nutrition, mass casualties, disability and mental health in conflict-affected populations

Importance of chronic and cross-cutting interventions

In recent years, typical areas of violent political conflict have changed, with greater numbers of higher-income, older and urban populations affected by conflict. These populations tend to be more vulnerable to chronic diseases, which require screening to detect and sustained medical attention to manage – both difficult to provide during conflict and among displaced populations. Conflict-affected populations in camps are living longer, due to improved living conditions and infectious disease control, and thus are increasingly susceptible to the chronic diseases traditionally affecting elderly populations. Additionally, recent experience has increased both capacity and confidence within the humanitarian community to provide long-term care (e.g. for HIV).

Long-term treatment for those affected by chronic infectious tuberculosis or hypertension may be disrupted during conflict. Approximately 15% of pregnant women will require some level of emergency care during delivery, irrespective of conflict. Nutrition interrelates with infectious disease control. Mass casualty responses address both violence-related and large-scale accidental injuries (e.g. landslides). Mental health and disability issues can pre-date or result from conflict violence. Thus, routine health care and support have an increasingly visible role in addressing the morbidity and mortality of conflict-affected populations.

Chronic non-infectious disease management

Definition

Chronic diseases are those that require long-term – sometimes life-long – management, often including a strict drug regimen and routine medical visits, and may or may not be curable. **Chronic infectious diseases**, such as HIV, are communicable but can be managed for years with the proper drug regimen. This section focuses on chronic *non-infectious* diseases, such as hypertension and diabetes, which require long-term management and sustained medical attention. Cancer is an increasingly important issue that is not always well-addressed in conflict-affected settings. Not all implementation agencies have the resources to address cancer. However, tansparent referral guidelines for secondary and tertiary care are crucial, particularly in middle-income counties.

Challenges of non-infectious diseases for conflict-affected populations

Age and income

In a trend beginning with the intra-state wars in the Balkans and Caucasus during the 1990s, conflicts are increasingly affecting older populations with higher incomes and better baseline health (Spiegel et al., 2010a). The profiles and health needs of these populations are different from those of the low-income, low-life-expectancy populations traditionally affected by conflict. Older, higher-income populations are less likely to suffer from diseases related to malnutrition or overcrowding, instead being more susceptible to non-infectious diseases commonly occurring in old age, such as hypertension and diabetes. The likelihood of contracting such diseases increases in conflict due to limited access to screening and medical care, compromised diets and increased stress levels. Moreover, support offered by humanitarian agencies to refugees and internally displaced persons (IDPs) is usually aimed at those aged 20–45, and the medical needs of those over age 45 are not readily met. Evidence indicates *current* chronic non-infectious conditions can be exacerbated in conflict settings because of physical and psychological stress and reduced access to medications. As today's displaced populations are older and more susceptible to either developing or exacerbating non-infectious chronic conditions, regular access to health services and medicine is particularly important. A study on mortality data from Kosovo found that chronic disease was the second leading cause of death during the conflict in 1998–9 (Spiegel and Salama, 2000). Exacerbation of existing conditions has also been found in post-disaster settings, as relief workers were less aware of non-infectious chronic disease needs (Chan and Sondorp, 2007). As infectious disease health services in camps continue to improve, residents are living longer and are increasingly vulnerable to non-infectious diseases associated with ageing.

Urban IDPs

As the world becomes increasingly urbanized, more forced migrants are displaced from rural to urban areas, often in search of the services and work opportunities more

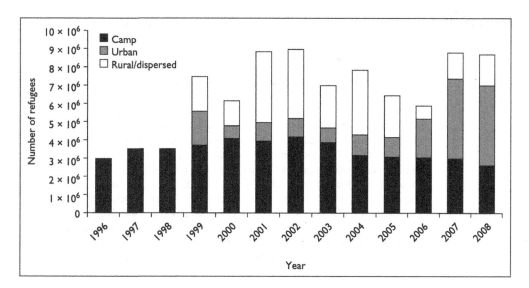

Figure 9.1 Numbers of refugees living in camp, urban or rural dispersed settings, 1996–2008
Source: (Spiegel et al., 2010a).

readily available in urban settings. As shown in Figure 9.1, the majority of refugees are now in urban areas, as opposed to in camps or rurally dispersed (Spiegel et al., 2010a).

In 2010, 90% of countries monitored by the Internal Displacement Monitoring Centre (IDMC) had migrants displaced by violence or conflict living in urban areas (International Displacement Monitoring Centre, 2010). In Columbia, for example, it is estimated that 90% of people who were forced to leave their homes in 2010 were displaced to urban areas (International Displacement Monitoring Centre, 2010). Despite the large number of IDPs in urban areas, humanitarian agencies tend to focus on IDPs in camps and rural areas as they are easier to access and manage. Unlike camp settings, IDPs in urban areas are dispersed and difficult to identify, making provision of health services challenging.

Post-conflict vulnerabilities

A relatively overlooked aspect of public health in conflict settings is the vulnerability of post-conflict areas to non-infectious chronic disease. Although, by definition, post-conflict areas are those in which violence has largely ceased, the health effects of conflict often endure. The psychological distress caused by conflict and displacement can lead to increased risk behaviours for non-infectious chronic disease, including alcohol or substance misuse and smoking (Roberts et al., 2012). These behaviours, along with decreased physical activity, are exacerbated by the urbanization commonly occurring in post-conflict settings and by tobacco, alcohol and food companies eager to profit from new markets (Roberts et al., 2012). Areas that have not yet emerged from conflict, but where conflict is 'frozen' or of low intensity, are also at high risk of increased non-infectious chronic diseases as the capacity to provide the necessarily complex and sustained care required is limited (e.g. the Caucasus).

Potential interventions to reduce the chronic disease burden among conflict-affected populations

Responding to the needs of conflict-affected populations susceptible to, or suffering from, chronic diseases often requires the sustained access to medical care that is especially challenging in conflict-affected areas where health systems are already strained (see Chapters 12 and 13 for more on health systems). Recognizing the challenges and importance of addressing chronic disease in conflict-affected populations, Spiegel et al. (2010a) advocated a systematic approach to prevention and management of chronic disease in conflict areas (Table 9.1). They recommend (i) identifying and registering as many prevalent cases of treatable chronic disease as possible when first responding to a conflict, (ii) providing simplified guidelines for home-based care, (iii) identifying effective ways of providing tuberculosis and HIV treatment that is less dependent on health system contact, (iv) training humanitarian staff in chronic disease care, and (v) anticipating increased costs associated with screening and long-term care. They recognize that treatment continuation in dispersed communities requires particular effort in conflict zones, and lulls in fighting should be used as opportunities to provide patients with home-based care and supplies.

Planning

Chronic disease management must be incorporated into disaster and post-disaster rehabilitation planning, and chronic diseases are now included in both the *Sphere Handbook* (Sphere, 2011) and *Health Cluster Guide* (IASC, 2009). Costs of chronic disease management must be included in disaster preparedness budgeting, prevalence of non-infectious disease cases should be determined, drug supplies stockpiled, and humanitarian staff sensitized to needs of chronic disease patients. Public health researchers can help by collecting more data on prevalence, determinants and effective prevention and management of chronic diseases in conflict settings.

Table 9.1 Recommendations for addressing chronic diseases in conflict settings

---

* Include systematic registration of prevalent cases of locally treatable chronic disease – at least tuberculosis, HIV/AIDS, diabetes, and cardiovascular disease – as a top priority during any emergency health response and develop rapid case identification methods (e.g. with key informant-driven or respondent-driven referral).
* Develop simplified home-based care guidelines for diabetes and heart disease and treatment kits for use in settings of insecurity and restricted health facility coverage.
* Investigate effectiveness and harm-to-benefit ratio of new, adherence-promoting ways to offer tuberculosis and AIDS treatment with reduced laboratory and health system contact needs, and safe treatment discontinuation strategies in case of permanent patient departure from programme catchment areas.
* Systematically include chronic disease care as part of public health training modules for humanitarian staff.
* Anticipate increased costs attributable to expensive tests and treatments, long disease duration, and specialist consultations in financial planning.

Source: Spiegel et al. (2010a).

Activity 9.1

Choose a specific chronic disease (e.g. hypertension). List the services necessary to manage this disease and potential challenges to providing these services for conflict-affected populations.

Sexual and reproductive health

Definitions

There is no universally recognized definition of sexual and reproductive health (SRH). The World Health Organization's working definitions describe a state of physical, mental and social well-being in relation to sexuality and reproductive processes, functions and system at all stages of life; that people are entitled to positive, respectful and safe sexuality, free of coercion, discrimination and violence, the capability to reproduce, and freedom to decide if, when and how often to do so. The key operational difference between *reproductive health* (RH) and SRH, that the latter includes rights, sexuality, and gender, has implications for service provision in conflict-affected areas. SRH addresses gender-based violence (GBV) explicitly, while reproductive health does not.

Challenges

Neglecting the SRH needs of conflict-affected populations not only goes against human rights and humanitarian principles but also has serious health and social consequences, including preventable maternal and infant deaths, unwanted pregnancies, unsafe abortions, sexual violence, and the spread of HIV and other sexually transmitted infections (STIs).

SRH interventions for conflict-affected populations

Considerable progress has been made in identifying and addressing the SRH needs of conflict-affected populations. Within the health cluster, SRH interventions for crisis-affected populations are implemented via the Minimum Initial Service Package (MISP). The MISP was developed by the Inter-Agency Working Group (IAWG) to provide for the most urgent SRH needs in acute crises. With its 12 related RH kits, the MISP is intended to provide personnel, supplies, equipment, initial activities, and planning for SRH service provision during acute crisis and the transition to longer-term comprehensive services. As shown in Figure 9.2, the MISP focuses on sexual violence, HIV transmission, and maternal and newborn health during acute crisis, with provisions for coordination and a transition to comprehensive services.

Coordination and transition to comprehensive services

Coordination of SRH activities (MISP Objective 1) can be complex as multiple agencies and sectors may be contributing at international, national and sub-national levels. In addition to health cluster leadership by WHO, a focal agency or person to coordinate MISP activities should be selected early in the crisis.

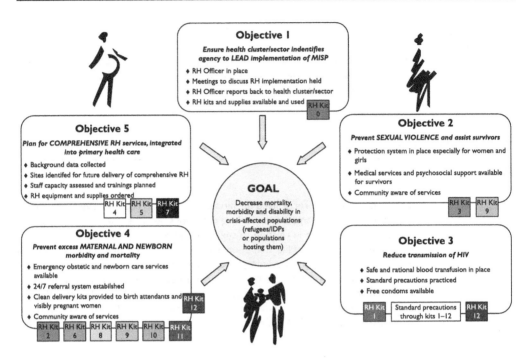

Figure 9.2 Minimum Initial Service Package for SRH in crises

Source: MISP online training course (RHRC, 2011).

The post-acute transition to comprehensive services (MISP Objective 5) should begin at the time the humanitarian community initiates longer-term (6–12-month) planning. Comprehensive SRH services must be integrated into funding and planning processes (e.g. consolidated appeals process, Common Humanitarian Action Plan) so that service provision (e.g. contraceptives other than condoms, gender-based violence, STI management) is not delayed unnecessarily.

Sexual violence

Considered a form of GBV, this is defined as any non-consensual sexual act (e.g. rape, attempted rape, sexual abuse) (RHRC, 2011). **Sexual violence** impacts a survivor's physical, mental, and social well-being, with consequences for the survivor's family and community (e.g. documented uses of rape as a strategy of war to control and humiliate communities) (Spiegel et al., 2011). UN Security Council Resolution 1325 entitles women and girls to protection from sexual violence in conflict settings. While male-on-female sexual violence is most reported, men and boys are also at risk, particularly in detention or torture settings (RHRC, 2011). Table 9.2 provides some health consequences of sexual violence.

Protecting affected populations from sexual violence and managing effects by ensuring availability and awareness of post-rape clinical services (MISP Objective 2) requires multi-sectoral cooperation. For example, UNHCR, as lead of the protection cluster, will provide input on protective interventions under the overall coordination of the

Table 9.2 Health consequences of sexual violence by any perpetrator

FATAL OUTCOMES	NON-FATAL OUTCOMES		
	Physical injuries and chronic conditions	Sexual and reproductive sequelae	Psychological and behavioural outcomes
• Femicide • Suicide • AIDS-related mortality • Maternal mortality	• Fractures • Abdominal/thoracic injuries • Chronic pain syndromes • Fibromyalgia • Permanent disability • Gastrointestinal disorders • Irritable bowel syndrome • Lacerations and abrasions • Ocular damage	• Gynaecological disorders • Pelvic inflammatory disease • Sexually transmitted infections, including HIV • Unwanted pregnancy • Pregnancy complications • Miscarriage/low birth weight • Sexual dysfunction • Unsafe abortion	• Depression and anxiety • Eating and sleeping disorders • Drug and alcohol abuse • Phobias and panel disorder • Poor self-esteem • Post-traumatic stress disorder (PTSD) • Psychosomatic disorders • Self-harm • Unsafe sexual behaviour

Source: Krug et al. (2002).

Camp Coordination and Camp Management cluster (e.g. location of latrines, provision of cooking fuel), while WHO is responsible for clinical interventions and UNFPA for gender-related issues (Figure 5.1).

Exposure to political violence is associated with increased odds of psychological, physical, sexual, and intimate-partner GBV (Clark et al., 2010). Thus, initiatives for post-acute or **chronic emergencies** should address a wider array of violence issues (e.g. domestic violence, early/forced marriage, female genital cutting, human trafficking, coerced prostitution).

Sexually-transmitted infections and HIV

MISP Objective 3 is intended to reduce HIV transmission though guaranteed and discrete access to condoms, safe blood transfusion, and ensuring respect for **standard precautions**. Standard infection control precautions require frequent hand-washing with soap, wearing gloves and protective clothing, and safe handling and disposal of sharps and biohazard waste. Initiatives for post-acute and chronic emergencies should include diagnosis and treatment of HIV and other STIs.

Maternal and newborn care

Of the approximately 4% in conflict-affected populations who will be pregnant, approximately 15% will experience an obstetric emergency (e.g. obstructed labour, eclampsia, sepsis, ectopic pregnancy, post-abortion complications). MISP Objective 4 intends to reduce excess maternal and neonatal mortality and morbidity through ensuring availability and accessibility of emergency obstetric and newborn care (EmONC) within health care institutions (Table 9.3), establishing referral systems from community to health centres and hospitals, and providing **clean delivery kits** to visibly pregnant women and birth attendants where facility access is unlikely.

Table 9.3 Basic versus comprehensive emergency obstetric and newborn care

Basic EmONC at all health facilities	Comprehensive EmONC at all hospitals
Ensure staff are skilled and have the resources to:	Ensure staff are skilled and have the resources to:
1. administer *parenteral* antibiotics	
2. administer *parenteral* uterotonics	*complete*
3. administer *parenteral* anticonvulsants	*tasks*
4. perform manual removal of the placenta	*1–7*
5. perform removal of retained products of conception	*plus*
6. perform assisted vaginal delivery	8. perform caesarean and laparotomy under anaesthesia
7. perform neonatal resuscitation	9. perform blood transfusions

Source: adapted from RHRC (2011).

Initiatives for post-acute and chronic emergencies include establishing antenatal care and training community midwives.

Activity 9.2

Briefly describe, using online or text resources, the shift from reproductive health to SRH approaches for conflict-affected populations. What significant policy changes underpin this shift?

Nutrition

Definitions and challenges

Nutrition is closely related to food security, the definition of which has evolved from simple availability in the 1970s to the rights-based statement at the 1996 World Food Summit that 'Food security exists when all people, at all times, have physical and economic access to sufficient, safe and nutritious food that meets their dietary needs and food preferences for an active and healthy life'.

Conflict often undermines household food security (Egal, 2006). Production may be disrupted, stores looted or destroyed, or livestock slaughtered, while insecurity and land-mines may prevent people growing crops. Many human-induced food emergencies are fuelled by conflict, often compounded by drought, flooding, or the AIDS pandemic. The population groups most nutritionally vulnerable during conflict are young children, pregnant and lactating women, older and disabled people, and those living with chronic illnesses such as HIV. Those who are already undernourished are much more likely to become ill and die, while those who are already ill are more likely to become undernourished.

Malnutrition develops when the body does not get the right amount of nutrients needed to maintain healthy function (i.e. over-nutrition, under-nutrition, micronutrient deficiencies). *Chronic malnutrition* reflects long-term nutrient deficiencies, or repeated episodes of disease or acute malnutrition, and presents as stunting. Stunting, relatively common in low-income countries, is not immediately life-threatening. *Acute malnutrition*

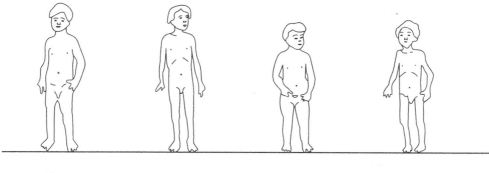

| Normal | Wasted | Stunted | Wasted and stunted |
| Normal weight and height | Thinner than normal | Shorter than normal | Thinner and shorter than normal |

Figure 9.3 Types of malnutrition
Source: B Fenn, LSHTM lecture (2012).

reflects current nutritional restrictions and presents as wasting or oedema. It is categorized as **severe acute malnutrition** (SAM), moderate acute malnutrition, or combined as **global acute malnutrition** (GAM). Clinical forms of SAM are *marasmus* (i.e. fat/muscle depletion and extreme thinness), *kwashiorkor* (i.e. fat/muscle depletion plus oedema), or combined as *marasmic-kwashiorkor*. SAM has a high mortality rate that is reversible with therapeutic feeding, thus requiring urgent intervention in crises. See Figure 9.3. Increasingly, the double burden of acute malnutrition and overweight/obesity must be addressed in conflict-affected settings, as this is occurring more frequently, particularly in middle-income countries.

Nutrition assessment

Nutrition assessment is used to determine crisis severity, identify those needing treatment referral, and inform planning, monitoring and evaluation. Different designs may be used depending on context (e.g. rapid nutrition assessment, survey, surveillance). Nutritional surveys allow calculation of malnutrition prevalence by selecting a representative sample of children (and increasingly adults) using simple random, systematic or cluster sampling (Young and Jaspers, 2006). Classification is based on standardized weight-for-height (WFH) ratio, bilateral oedema, or **mid-upper arm circumference** (MUAC) in children aged 6–59 months, or Body Mass Index (BMI) in adults. Use of absolute thresholds to determine severity is common among agencies though debated by experts. Both SAM and GAM (threshold 15–20% depending on agency) are sensitive crisis indicators preceding mortality rate increases, and should be measured regularly.

Activity 9.3

Calculate your BMI by dividing you weight in kilograms by the square of your height in metres, and compare it to Table 9.4. Then, using online or print resources, identify potential challenges in using standardized WFH, MUAC and BMI for assessment.

Table 9.4 Estimating adult nutrition level using BMI

Type & level of malnutrition	BMI range (kg/m²)
Obese	30.0+
Overweight	25.0–29.9
Normal	18.5–24.9
CED* Mild	17.0–18.4
CED Moderate	16.0–16.9
CED Severe	<16.0

* Chronic Energy Deficiency.

Clinical signs of under-nutrition and changes in anthropometric measurements are late indicators for intervention. Assessing the determinants of nutrition, and effects of conflict on affected population and vulnerable groups, associated with simple indicators of food consumption (e.g. dietary diversity scores, predicted energy intake scores) that are sensitive in both crisis and rehabilitation, may provide a better basis for action (NutritionWorks, 2011).

Nutrition interventions

Both severe and moderate malnutrition are treatable through nutritional rehabilitation programmes. Community-based therapeutic care is increasingly the consensus approach, whereby only severely malnourished children with serious infections are treated on an inpatient basis and the rest receive home-based care (Checchi et al., 2007). In recent years, **community-based management of severe malnutrition**, made possible through the use of **ready-to-use therapeutic food**, has increased coverage beyond levels achievable with centre-based programmes.

Responses should aim to prevent as well as treat under-nutrition (Van Ommeren and Tol, 2011). During and after conflicts, protecting the nutritional status of affected populations is crucial. Food aid and **nutritional rehabilitation** are essential to preserving lives in the short run, but cannot provide lasting solutions unless combined with interventions addressing structural health and environmental issues, such as livelihood support (Egal, 2006).

Under-nutrition does not result simply from lack of food but from a complex combination of environmental, social and political factors affecting populations and households; thus a broad-based consensus approach is required to address it. UNICEF is the lead agency for the global nutrition cluster, which focuses on coordination, resource mobilization, and policy guidelines.

Mass casualty management

Defining the problem

Injuries are a significant public health challenge, accounting for 17% of the adult global burden of disease, and present a particular challenge in resource-limited conflict settings where mass events (e.g. explosions) can rapidly overwhelm existing resources and expertise. In conflict settings with few alternative health services, any health facility may be confronted with a major incident involving mass casualties. Major incidents are defined as any situation where field resources are suddenly overwhelmed, and are classified as **compounded** when accompanied by a loss of existing infrastructure and **uncompensated** when additional external resources are required (Redmond et al., 2005). Contingency planning and awareness of mass casualty management are therefore necessary for all health facilities in areas prone to major incidents (Ryan et al., 2002).

Emergency preparedness and incident response

Planning, preparation and training need to involve all members of the health care facility, from medics, logisticians and administrators to drivers and security guards. The *all-hazard* strategy for any major incident focuses planning on the seven key components of command and control, safety, communication, assessment, triage, treatment and transport of the injured (CSCATTT). The initial priority, in major incidents occurring away from health facilities, is rapid assessment and evacuation. This may involve deployment of mobile medical teams, for which necessary equipment and staff should be considered in advance and contact lists of key personnel regularly updated.

Following a mass casualty incident, the facility is likely to receive a sudden surge in patients, relatives, authorities and general public, potentially exacerbating initial chaos. It is useful to pre-designate separate coordinators for medical and administrative domains to jointly control initial response, and designate specific areas for reassessment on arrival, treatment zones according to severity of injury, access to emergency stock, and temporary storage of the dead. A clear communications structure should be agreed for potential insecurity following a major incident and dealing with media interest.

Triage and medical assessment

Triage, the key activity in mass casualty management, is the continuous process of rapidly assessing the injured to *do the most for the most*. The universal colour-coding system is useful for all involved in major incident planning, to assist patient flow and identify sickest patients. A rapid, initial **triage sieve** is conducted at the scene by trained personnel. This involves assessment of breathing rate, skin perfusion and mobility, and assigning a colour-coded tag around the patient's neck for easy identification and rapid transport to the appropriate location (see Table 9.5).

Table 9.5 Triage sieve categories

Priority	Treatment required	Colour designation
P1	Immediate/life-threatening	Red
P2	Urgent	Yellow
P3	Delayed	Green
P4	Dead	White

Source: J Pallett, 2012.

A more detailed assessment is performed on arrival at a designated casualty clearing station in the health facility. A **triage sort** is conducted and an *injury severity score* calculated once the patient is stabilized. One of the hardest tasks for those involved in triage in resource-limited environments is identifying patients most likely to benefit from immediately available interventions and not diverting limited resources to those with severe and complex injuries for whom longer-term management will not be available and treatment ultimately futile. Triage is therefore usually carried out by the most senior medical officer available, but ethical issues around rationing remain particularly when considering human rights and humanitarian law (Domres et al., 2001).

Injury patterns and treatment

While treatment of the main causes of excess mortality and morbidity (e.g. infectious diseases, malnutrition) can be anticipated following conflict-caused crises, the wide spectrum of injuries, varying levels of expertise, and resources required for successful management present considerable challenges. The approach to all injuries follows *advanced trauma life support* principles involving sequential steps known as C-ABC, consisting of controlling major haemorrhage, ensuring an airway, and assessing breathing and circulation (Advanced Life Support Group, 2002; Driscoll et al., 2000). This initial procedure needs to be conducted in the initial **golden hour** following injury when life-saving treatment is most effective.

Agencies responding to mass casualty events need to consider the logistics of providing surgery, which often involves specialized equipment, radiology imaging, supply chain, blood transfusion, anaesthetic support, sterilization, and prolonged rehabilitation with psychological support. However, 85–90% of mass casualty injuries are minor and can be treated with minimal resources (e.g. dressings, painkillers, antibiotics) provided in most health care facilities.

Sustainability

During crises in resource-limited settings, difficult decisions must often be made regarding resource allocation. For example, following explosions or natural disasters, severe crush injuries and open limb fractures are encountered that can require intensive resources (e.g. kidney replacement, limb reconstruction). Explicit consideration must be given to the opportunity costs of undertaking such interventions given the lack of basic health care and the need for subsequent long-term rehabilitation that relief agencies cannot often assure. The WHO Essential Trauma Care project provides valuable guidance on standards of trauma care for developing countries (WHO, 2009).

Disability

Definition and challenges

The UN Convention on the Rights of Persons with Disabilities describes disability as 'an evolving concept [that] results from the interaction between persons with impairments and attitudinal and environmental barriers that hinders their full and effective participation in society on an equal basis with others'. Article 1 of the Convention states that persons with disabilities include 'those who have long-term physical, mental, intellectual or sensory impairments which in interaction with various barriers may hinder their full and effective participation in society on an equal basis with others'.

WHO estimates that 7–10% of the world's population, including 3 million displaced persons, live with some form of disability (Reilly, 2008). Structural changes during conflict (e.g. exposure to violence, loss of social support or income, changes in physical infrastructure, political exclusion) can increase the vulnerability of those with pre-existing disabilities, while conflict-related injuries (e.g. landmines, bullets) can increase the numbers living with disabilities.

The Convention came into force in May 2008, though most agencies have been slow to adopt its rights-based approaches to disability policy and practice (Lang et al., 2011). Several assumptions contribute, particularly in conflict-affected settings. First, disability issues may not be considered until they become obvious (e.g. landmine survivors, large populations with disabilities). Second, humanitarian actors may believe they lack the skills to address the special needs of persons with disabilities, preferring to leave interventions to 'disability specialists'. Third, stigma and prejudice can complicate the mainstreaming of persons with disabilities into humanitarian programmes. Although the **medical model of disability** has been abandoned, it may influence medical staff and policy-makers.

Disability interventions

Most disability interventions in conflict-affected settings are conducted by a few major international NGOs and agencies (e.g. Christian Blind Mission, Handicap International, ICRC rehabilitation programme) with the support of local NGOs and **disabled people's organizations**. These specialist organizations implement programmes, by order of importance, in: physical rehabilitation, including physiotherapy and orthopaedic services; special education; and **community-based rehabilitation (CBR)**, based on the WHO CBR matrix (WHO et al., 2010). Some non-specialist NGOs (e.g. Swedish Committee of Afghanistan) include disabled people in their programmes or develop disability programmes. Key interventions include the following:

- *Assistive devices and technologies.* Prostheses, mobility aides, hearing and visual aids enable people with disabilities in conflict-affected settings to live more independently.
- *Special education.* Ideally, most students with disabilities can be provided with the support to participate in mainstream schools.
- *Rehabilitation.* To enable people with disabilities to reach and maintain optimal physical, sensory, intellectual, psychological and social function, this encompasses rehabilitative medical care; physical, psychological, speech, and occupational therapies; and CBR (i.e. rehabilitation, equalization of opportunity, poverty reduction, social inclusion).
- *Disability mainstreaming.* Non-disabled beneficiaries may be reluctant to participate in the same programmes as persons with disabilities, fearing bad luck or disease linked to the impairment. Persons with disabilities are often reluctant to participate, fearing bullying and rejection. Humanitarian actors may lack adequate tools to achieve inclusion. Decision-makers may consider mainstreaming too complex and expensive in resource-constrained settings. However, mainstreaming is the most cost-effective and least stigmatizing way to address the needs of persons with disabilities. While technical

assistance is needed for interventions such as demining, physical rehabilitation or special education, non-specialist agencies providing vocational training, economic support and infrastructure can include disabled people with minimal adaptation (Sphere, 2011).

Disabled people are at risk of poverty and exclusion, especially in conflict and post-conflict settings, and interventions and resources remain limited. While not intrinsically vulnerable, potential vulnerability is created for those with disabilities if conflict is exacerbated by lack of access to services, information and support.

Mental health

Definitions

Mental disorders constitute an important and growing part of the global burden of disease, estimated at 27% in high-income and 9% in low-income countries in 2005 and expected to rise to 29% and 11% in 2030 (Prince et al., 2007). However, mental health is more than the absence of mental disorder, encompassing well-being and social functioning. Therefore, the composite term mental health and psychosocial problems encompasses three broad categories of non-disordered distress, common mental disorders and severe mental disorders.

Non-disordered distress can be caused by violence, substance use, reaction to war and repression, socioeconomic difficulties, and marginalization (e.g. widows, orphans, people with disabilities). Psychosocial problems usually manifest as individual social dysfunction and/or interpersonal problems with family or social networks, but may also lead to symptoms of mental disorders in people with pre-existing vulnerabilities. Individuals with unstable or insufficient social networks are particularly at risk (e.g. children experiencing disrupted nurturing, women overburdened with family responsibilities or experiencing domestic violence).

Common mental disorders include mild and moderate depression and anxiety disorders, substance abuse, and moderate post-traumatic stress disorder. The aetiology of these disorders is strongly connected to social factors.

Severe mental disorders include psychosis, bipolar disorder, and severe depression. People with these disorders have typical symptoms and may be labelled mentally ill. Aetiology is largely unknown, including genetic and developmental factors, but onset and course are significantly influenced by contextual factors.

Challenges

In acute and chronic emergencies the prevalence of mental distress and disorders rises (Miller and Rasmussen, 2010). Generally, the prevalence of severe mental disorders rises due to disruption of protective social mechanisms and collapse of care systems, leading to relapses in previously stable and controlled disorders. The prevalence of common mental disorders usually more than doubles, due to increased causal factors including loss, traumatic events, and breakdown of social support structures. Particularly during social upheaval and conflict, it is challenging to distinguish between mental disorders and 'non-disordered distress'. The extent of observed increases in mental disorder and distress frequency is dependent on factors including: (i) time since the emergency, (ii) assessment methods, (iii) sociocultural factors underpinning coping

Table 9.6 WHO projections of psychological distress and mental disorders in adult emergency-affected populations

	BEFORE EMERGENCY: 12-month prevalence (median across countries and across level of exposure to adversity)[a]	AFTER EMERGENCY: 12-month prevalence (median across countries and across level of exposure to adversity)
Severe mental disorder	2–3%	3–4%
Mild or moderate mental disorder	10%	15–20%
'Normal' distress/other psychological reactions (no disorder)	No estimate	Large percentage

Source: Van Ommeren and Tol (2011).

[a] Assumed baseline rates are the median rates across countries as observed in the World Mental Health Survey 2000.

strategies and community social support, and (iv) previous and current crisis exposure (Table 9.6).

Interventions

The aftermath of collective violence is characterized by both increased needs and severe shortages of resources to address these needs. There is limited evidence on the effectiveness of mental health and psychosocial support after conflicts, but there is growing consensus that post-conflict mental and psychosocial issues should be addressed through integrated, multi-layered support aimed at fostering self-help and integrating care within existing health and social systems (Tol et al., 2011; IASC, 2007).

In conflict-affected settings, specialized mental health care systems are likely to be overwhelmed by the massive mental health needs of the population. Minimum levels of care for people with severe mental disorders can best be reached by integrating mental health into the general health care system. A useful clinical tool to assist non-specialist health workers is the *mhGAP Intervention Guide for Mental, Neurological and Substance Use Disorders in Non-specialized Health Settings* (WHO, 2010a). This guide provides clinical decision-making protocols and guidance for managing priority conditions (i.e. depression, psychosis, bipolar disorders, epilepsy, developmental and behavioural disorders in children and adolescents, dementia, alcohol use disorders, drug use disorders, self-harm/suicide, and other significant emotional or medically unexplained complaints). Treatment for common mental disorders, such as depression, should not be reduced to pharmacological interventions alone. It is critically important to combine medical and social interventions, foster intersectoral collaboration and promote the inclusion of capacity building and policy development. (Ventevogel et al., 2012).

Key to improving mental health care in conflict-affected communities is looking beyond narrowly defined health systems. Mental disorders and poverty interact in a negative cycle, and to break this, interventions need to address both social causes of mental disorders and the economic deprivation and social marginalization that are a consequence of mental disorders (Lund et al., 2011). Improving mental health of conflict-affected populations should integrate mental health in general social policies to improve population well-being. The psychosocial distress of survivors of collective violence can largely be alleviated through community-based approaches that strengthen capacities to deal with distress and adversity, such as women's support groups; child-friendly spaces, and livelihood support (Wessells and van Ommeren, 2008).

Post-conflict mental health programmes may, paradoxically, provide opportunities for long-term structural improvements if they build local capacity and sustainable systems of mental health care. For example, in Sri Lanka, Afghanistan and Liberia increased public awareness of mental health problems, and availability of significant health system reconstruction funding, led to significant mental health care reforms (Ventevogel et al., 2011).

Conclusions

This chapter discusses long-term and cross-cutting issues for consideration when developing and implementing health interventions for conflict-affected populations. The following chapter discusses monitoring and evaluation.

Feedback on Activities

Feedback on Activity 9.1

If you use the example of hypertension, you may have a similar list to the following:

Service	Challenges in conflict-affected populations
Regular BP checks	• Instability may reduce access to health staff
Adherence to BP-lowering medication	• Supply chain may be disrupted
Advice on diet/lifestyle	• Health staff may be difficult to access • Advice may be impractical given ongoing instability

Feedback on Activity 9.2

You may have considered some of the following. RH is health-based and focuses on 'moral' targets (e.g. married women) or the whole population. SRH is rights-based, advocating rights of access for all groups including 'high-risk' targets (e.g. sex workers, men who have sex with men), and explicitly includes GBV issues. Key policies and documents underpinning sexual and reproductive rights include the following:

- Universal Declaration of Human Rights (1948);
- International Covenant on Civil and Political Rights (1966);
- Convention on the Elimination of All Forms of Discrimination against Women (1972);
- Convention on the Rights of the Child (1989), which, for example, rejected child marriage and sexual abuse;
- International Conference on Population and Development (ICPD) Programme of Action (1994), in which the international community first agreed a broad

definition of reproductive health and rights and acknowledged refugees as an underserved group;
- Beijing Declaration (1995), of which paragraph 96 extended the definition of reproductive rights to cover sexuality;
- Commission on Human Rights, Resolution 2003/28 (2003).

Agencies have long addressed sexuality and reproduction, initially largely negatively through population control programmes or scare tactics for HIV prevention. Prior to the ICPD, there was little cohesive action, and the SRH needs of conflict-affected populations were not considered in international policy frameworks. The large number of rapes during the Bosnia crisis focused global attention on sexual health and rights among conflict-affected populations. More positive current approaches consider realization of sexual rights as crucial for social justice.

Feedback on Activity 9.3

If you are a healthy adult, it is unlikely your BMI will be within the CED categories. When reviewing nutritional indicators, you may have noted that WFH is advised for surveys, but requires some technical knowledge to calculate. MUAC is relatively easy, and useful for determining eligibility for therapeutic feeding, but can be done incorrectly. BMI is not particularly sensitive, but there is currently no methodologically simpler alternative for adults and adolescents in resource-constrained conflict settings.

10

Monitoring and evaluation

Peter Giesen

Overview

The aim of this chapter is to provide an overview of project monitoring and evaluation related to conflict-affected settings. Concepts and frameworks from programme management are used to explore monitoring and evaluation concepts, values, tools, methodologies and adaptations required in conflict settings.

Learning outcomes

After completing this chapter you should be able to:

- describe reasons for project monitoring and evaluation in crises
- identify key steps and tools in the logical framework approach to project monitoring and evaluation
- consider conflict-specific aspects of monitoring and the logical framework approach
- discuss evaluation of humanitarian health interventions

Monitoring and evaluation in crises

Reasons and challenges

The challenges to monitoring and evaluating health interventions in conflict situations are similar to those in delivery of the services themselves. Like service delivery, data collection requires presence on the ground and focuses on population with specific needs in specific circumstances. Characteristics to be considered include fluid populations, social and cultural dislocation, systems collapse, lack of accountability, and conflict-related health problems.

Humanitarian activities often occur as programmes, whereby an agency implements a specific set of interventions based on the humanitarian needs of a population and influenced by the agency's mandate, capacities and resources. The agency and its funders will want to know if it has achieved what it set out to do, if it can account for resources used, and what lessons can be learned. A **project cycle** relates planning activities, implementation, monitoring and evaluation. A **logical framework** enables rational planning of activities that can be monitored and evaluated.

Definitions

This chapter uses monitoring and evaluation terminology as defined in the OECD/DAC monitoring and evaluation glossary, because it is comprehensive, well researched and widely used (OECD/DAC, 2002). While *programmes* are larger and usually last longer than *projects*, the terms can be considered interchangeably in this chapter. Donors increasingly require accountability for results. As monitoring and evaluation include donor accountability, the glossary has the added advantage of consistency with donor terminology.

OECD/DAC defines *monitoring* as a continuing function, using systematic data collection on specified indicators, to provide the management and main stakeholders of an ongoing intervention with indications of the extent of progress and achievement of objectives and progress in the use of allocated funds. Several key elements are included.

First, monitoring is defined as a *continuing* process, implying ongoing access to populations while monitoring outcomes. Access to conflict-affected populations cannot be guaranteed, raising potential challenges.

Second, monitoring provides *management* with information, so management should be included when designing protocols and determining the information required to steer the programme (e.g. how much information and how often). This can guide an efficient and purpose-focused monitoring protocol, providing user-friendly and user-focused management information, without increasing bureaucracy. This is particularly important in conflict situations, where programmes need to save lives and information gathering needs to be in the service of this central objective.

Third, monitoring provides information for other *stakeholders* (e.g. donors, government officials). This may introduce dilemmas, as each stakeholder may want different information. To avoid burdensome data collection in environments where life-saving activities take priority, it is imperative for stakeholders to agree a monitoring protocol requiring minimum essential data requirements. This has consequences for the number of indicators and feasibility of data collection in conflict settings.

OECD/DAC defines *evaluation* as the systematic and objective assessment of an ongoing or completed project, programme or policy, including design, implementation and results. The phrase *systematic and objective* implies methodological discipline, but conflict can cause the collapse of systems and create significant challenges to evaluation design and implementation. Monitoring and evaluation are complementary. During evaluation, as much monitoring data is used as possible. In monitoring, emphasis is on process and results, while evaluation is used to provide insight into the relationships between results, outcomes and impact.

The logical framework approach

The project cycle

Since monitoring is defined in the context of project management, the project cycle (Figure 10.1) is a widely used project management conceptualization tool that shows how monitoring and evaluation relate to planning, implementation and assessment.

Logical framework approach

Monitoring focuses on *planned* objectives, but where do these objectives come from? Who determines them and what process defines them? The most widely used approach to setting objectives is *objectives-oriented project planning* (OOPP) using a

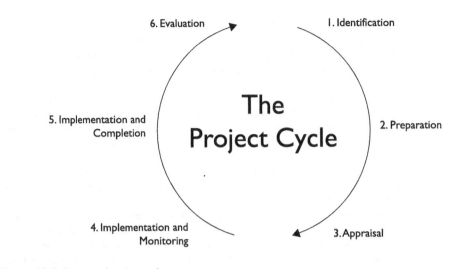

Figure 10.1 Project planning cycle

logical framework (logframe). This eight-step team-building and planning process, developed by Leon Rosenberg for the US Agency for International Development (USAID) in 1969, involves:

(1) brainstorming problems facing the conflict-affected population;
(2) developing a *problem tree*, linking problems in a cause-and-effect flowchart;
(3) conversion into an *objective tree* by redefining problems into achieved positive results;
(4) clustering *in* results the project team wants to address, and clustering *out* results that are responsibilities of other actors;
(5) providing *intervention logic* by moving clusters into objectives and assumptions (or risks) columns, leaving the cause-and-effect hierarchy from the problem tree intact;
(6) developing *indicators* and *means of verification* (MoV) through data collection.

This process can be illustrated with a simplified example from a project workshop on HIV in the conflict-affected southern Caucasus.

Step 1: Brainstorming. The project team freely exchanges ideas, without any preconceived structure, about problems facing the conflict-affected population. Knowing they will address HIV, they focus on related issues, and come up with the following list:

• people die from AIDS
• people contract the virus
• poor attitudes within the health system
• people have unsafe sex
• treatment in health facilities is poor

- people are not aware of the risks
- people do not use condoms
- few resources
- drug users share needles
- blood screening in health facilities is poor

Step 2: Problem tree. The team links brainstormed problems together by cause and effect, resulting in a problem tree (Figure 10.2).

Step 3: Conversion. The team converts the problems in the tree into positive and achieved changes, leaving all the interrelationships intact (Figure 10.3).

Step 4: Clustering. The team decides, based on organizational policy and available resources (Figure 10.4), the problems it will address with direct activities (left-hand ellipse) and those that should be addressed by other actors (right-hand ellipse).

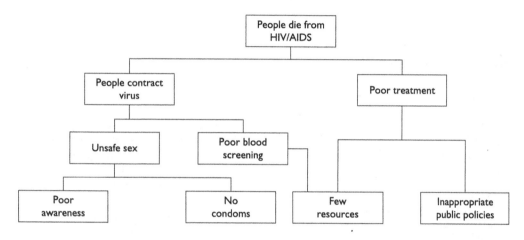

Figure 10.2 Problem tree example

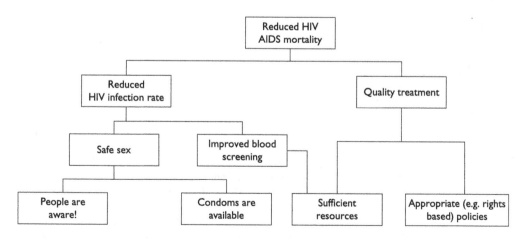

Figure 10.3 Objective tree example

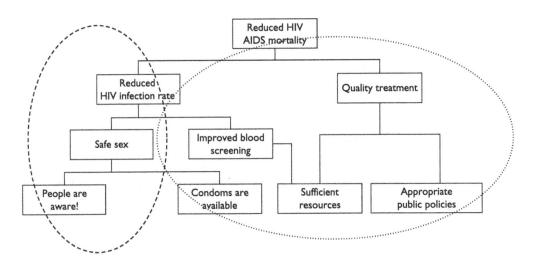

Figure 10.4 Clustering example

Objectives *Overall*	Indicators	Sources of Verification	Advocacy (responsibilities of others)
Reduced AIDS mortality			Quality treatment (incl. drugs)
Project Purpose Reduced HIV infection rate **= IMPACT**			Improved blood screening Appropriate attitudes in health system
Specific Objective People have safe sex **= OUTCOME**			Condoms available
Activities Awareness campaign **= OUTPUT**			Sufficient resources

Figure 10.5 Intervention logic example

> *Step 5: Intervention logic.* The team places clustered in results into the left-hand column of a logframe and what they clustered out into the right-hand column. The resulting intervention logic (Figure 10.5), allows the right-hand column to serve as an advocacy checklist. Next, the team checks its logic (Figure 10.6), using the same cause-and-effect approach as for building the problem tree (e.g. is it true that people will have safe sex if the project manages to increase awareness while other parties make condoms available?).

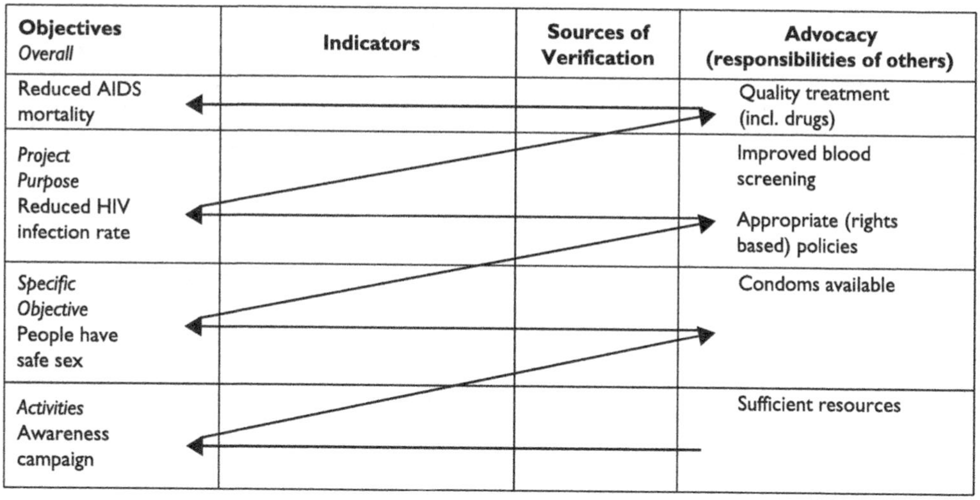

Objectives *Overall*	Indicators	Sources of Verification	Advocacy (responsibilities of others)
Reduced AIDS mortality			Quality treatment (incl. drugs)
Project *Purpose* Reduced HIV infection rate			Improved blood screening Appropriate (rights based) policies
Specific *Objective* People have safe sex			Condoms available
Activities Awareness campaign			Sufficient resources

Figure 10.6 Intervention logic checking example

Table 10.1 SMART indicators

S	Specific	It should refer to a specific area or target population.
M	Measurable	It should be scorable on a scale, either quantitatively or qualitatively, thus requiring a target and/or baseline (e.g. mortality reduced by 15% from baseline).
A	Achievable	It should be feasible within time-frame and budget (e.g. is it too ambitious?). Is a 15% reduction a feasible target, given the timeline and nature and complexity of the problems?
R	Relevant	It should be an essential indicator. Are other indicators more essential?
	Reliable	If different people collect the same information, they should obtain the same result.
T	Time-bound	It should state the time by which you expect to achieve change, and relates to achievability (e.g. within 3 years from project start).

Source: Adapted from Doran (1981).

Step 6: Indicators and MoV. Once satisfied with its logic, the team develops indicators adapted from reliable sources. For example, Sphere project indicators are often used in humanitarian settings (Sphere, 2011). Means of verification indicate either the actor who will provide data, or the data to be used if the team is collecting it. The team ensures that indicators are SMART (Table 10.1). This process of objectives-oriented project planning results in a logframe (Figure 10.7). The right-hand column is labelled 'advocacy', rather than 'assumptions' as is often used, because it is assumed not only that others will complete necessary interventions, but also that project managers can take an active role in advocating for those necessary interventions to be conducted.

Objectives *Overall*	Indicators (NL)	Sources of Verification	Advocacy (responsibilities of others)
Reduced AIDS mortality	<100/year by 2010	UNAIDS	Quality treatment (incl. drugs)
Impact Reduced HIV infection rate	<18,000 by 2010	UNAIDS	Improved blood screening Appropriate (rights based) policiies
Outcome People have safe sex	Condoms sales up	Industry/ import figures	Condoms available
Output Awareness campaign	Inputs	Budget	Sufficient resources

Figure 10.7 Logical framework example

Activity 10.1

You have been asked to help a team of government and international NGO malaria experts develop a logframe for a control project in County X, a remote area affected by chronic low-level conflict. Their brainstorming contributed the following information: the malaria-specific mortality rate in County X is presumed to be 15.4 per thousand person-years; the population is approximately 200,000; 20% of the population currently uses untreated mosquito nets; the local health centres have been destroyed and the government supply chain is disrupted; private sector suppliers can access most areas of County X and there is an active weekly market. Using this information, construct a simple logframe, using the steps outlined in the section above.

Conflict-specific challenges of the logframe approach

Criticism of the logframe approach for conflict settings

The concepts and tools of the logframe approach apply equally in humanitarian and more stable development contexts. Common criticisms of the logframe approach include rigidity, not reflecting reality, and the need for stability. However, logframes remain a broadly recognized and useful tool for structuring implementation, monitoring and evaluation.

Rigidity

It is tempting to reject the linear cause-and-effect nature of the problem tree when agency projects focus on solving complex social problems in unstable conflict-affected settings. Cause and effect are not easily identifiable. Factors may be mutually reinforcing rather than causal. For example, the relationships between conflict, malnutrition and viral infection, when considering an HIV project in a conflict-affected area, are not only linear. Conflict may displace people, undermine food security and cause nutritional status to deteriorate. Poor food security may contribute to further escalation of the conflict. Poor nutritional status may cause higher susceptibility to viral infections, contributing to deteriorating nutritional status through immobilization and loss of appetite. These demonstrate mutually reinforcing rather than causal relationships and should be noted as such where possible in the problem tree.

Lacking reality

Logframes may not accurately represent the true nature of problems confronting the population, and users must realize that a problem tree is a conceptual model and not reality. All models underlying monitoring protocols are based on certain assumptions. The more planning participants are connected with field realities, the more likely their assumptions will approximate reality, enabling the logframe to be a useful monitoring tool for the real situation in the field.

Requiring stability

Creating a logframe-based monitoring and evaluation framework assumes generally stable conditions during implementation and monitoring at least. However, in conflict-affected areas, situations may rapidly destabilize and projects consequently must adapt to remain relevant. Time pressures may preclude subsequent formal planning exercises. While the need for flexibility and responsiveness under these conditions is apparent, it creates difficulties for effective project monitoring and evaluation. To address this, evaluators of humanitarian projects may construct a logframe retrospectively to enable comparison of intended and actual results.

General monitoring challenges in conflict-affected settings

Challenges complicating project monitoring in conflict-affected areas include population mobility, unreliable or missing data, and accountability.

Mobility

People exposed to conflict, with limited protection, may choose self-displacement as a survival strategy or be forcibly displaced by belligerents or other actors (e.g. move from home to a camp, seek protection in another country). Camps and transitional settlements are sometimes relocated due to changing protection or service delivery requirements. Normal data collection techniques are often inadequate for conflict-affected populations. Counting mobile populations is not easy, so even the most basic information is not always available. Satellite imagery and other remote estimation methods may help, but crude data need to be verified through assessment on the ground, and mobile phone technology plays a greater role. Monitoring health problems of mobile conflict-affected populations becomes additionally challenging when multiple contacts are required (e.g. therapeutic feeding). Monitoring the nutritional status of children under age 5 can only occur when the situation has stabilized sufficiently to allow targeted interventions and data collection.

During acute stages of conflict, monitoring may not be possible and alternative, cruder methodologies may be applied. Access to populations may be limited, as belligerents have other priorities than population health and may be anxious about collection of social or health-related data from populations for whom they are responsible. Monitoring the health of mobile conflict-affected populations requires adaptation of indicators and data collection, preferably in a way that reflects realistic outcomes. Feasibility of data collection is an important consideration. There is no benefit in formulating indicators for which data cannot be collected due to insecurity or lack of consistent access.

Unreliable or missing data

In conflict-affected areas, critical shortages of reliable quantitative data can challenge evidence-based programming. Conflict can cause the collapse of national and sub-national health system infrastructure, leaving populations without vital services and monitors without routinely collected data. Military operations may hamper data collection, due to security risks to health care providers and data collectors. The social chaos and turmoil caused by conflict have profound impacts on public health information systems, which often remain dysfunctional long after conflict has formally ended. Health systems generate important quantitative data, and system disruptions often mean that decision-makers become dependent on qualitative information. Experience has shown that in conflict situations data reliability sharply decreases beyond the output level. It is therefore advisable to choose a very limited number of measurable outcome indicators and opt for more qualitative approaches. While valid for decision-making and evaluation under constrained circumstances, operational data may not be robust enough to contribute to the evidence base, making operational data collection and analysis different from research.

Responsibility and accountability

Three types of humanitarian responsibilities are legal, technical and moral. The Geneva Conventions stipulate responsibilities for the well-being, including health, of conflict-affected populations. Evaluations with a strong accountability agenda require outcomes that are referenced to formal responsibilities for service delivery and protection. Technical references include Sphere standards and agency-specific indicators (e.g. MSF clinical guidelines). These standards measure outcomes of collective action and, unlike output indicators, are not suitable for single agency accountability.

The humanitarian charter specifies conditions under which the Sphere standards are valid, including that all actors uphold their formal responsibilities to affected populations (Sphere, 2011). However, these conditions may not prevail in humanitarian crises, as it is precisely the lack of accountability and consideration for the needs of the population that contributed to initiation of conflict.

Evaluation of humanitarian interventions

Evaluation has received increasing attention in recent years, in terms of learning and accountability. The end-of-project evaluation is probably the most routine form of humanitarian evaluation, with a mix of learning and accountability objectives. While monitoring is a routine process of data collection for management and reporting, evaluation is intended to be strategic.

Evaluation approaches

While all evaluation must encompass beneficiary perspectives, some general evaluation approaches and types include learning, accountability, joint and real-time.

Learning evaluation

This is usually scoped to study specific issues on the strategic agenda of the programming agency. In the evaluation terms of reference these issues are usually listed in the *key questions* section. For example, an NGO may wish to learn about its capacity to implement a particular technical project in which it has recently acquired experience (e.g. Oxfam commissioned several evaluations of its food security projects, MSF commissioned three comparative evaluations of exit strategies, IFRC commissioned three real-time evaluations of the impact of its decentralization in the Philippines, Indonesia, Haiti and Pakistan).

Accountability evaluation

The process is often driven by the donor and expectations that the report will focus on the extent to which the project contributes to a wider policy intention. For example, the Dutch government actively pursues a stabilization agenda for fragile states, so Netherlands-based agencies receiving Dutch humanitarian funding must demonstrate the extent to which projects have both saved lives and contributed to the donor agenda (e.g. improvements in community-level governance, economic sustainability for disarmed combatants improved gender relations).

Joint evaluation

Networks such as ALNAP (www.alnap.co.uk) and national evaluation associations (e.g. American Evaluation Society, African Evaluation Society) have fuelled important debates about the quality and utility of evaluations. The Joint Evaluation of Emergency Assistance to Rwanda (JEEAR) and the Tsunami Evaluation Coalition (TEC) are important examples of joint evaluations and collaboration at sector level and have generated much debate, giving rise to newly emerging humanitarian agendas.

Real-time evaluation

Real-time evaluations (RTEs) are a recently developed approach that emerged when *ex-post evaluations* (i.e. implemented after an intervention) had difficulties finding key stakeholders and decision-makers to interview, due to high staff turnover once the crisis intervention ended. RTEs are intended to provide managers with strategic information during operations that monitoring alone cannot provide.

Most evaluations include both learning and accountability, though emphasis varies. If the focus is organizational learning, evaluations are largely internal as learning increases with high trust levels and credibility of peer evaluators. *Self-evaluation* is perhaps the most radical example of internal learning evaluation. In contrast, accountability evaluations are generally implemented by external specialists, using professional standards or donor policy frameworks (e.g. *inspection, audit*).

Evaluating humanitarian health interventions

Regardless of the type of evaluation, several commonalities characterize evaluation of humanitarian health interventions. During acute conflict, interventions tend to be short and focused on saving lives. Quantifiable indicators may only be suitable at output level (e.g. number of condoms distributed), as outcomes and impact are difficult to quantify. Short project duration and high staff turnover during acute conflict indicate lighter, internally managed evaluations (e.g. World Vision's *after action workshops*, MSF's self-evaluations), organized as one-day workshops and sometimes facilitated by an external consultant.

Project evaluations in conflict-affected settings are more dependent on qualitative data than those in stable settings. Despite this, some donors call for evidence-based programming and evaluation in conflict settings, which, given the lack of reliable outcome and impact data, is perhaps difficult to justify. Robertson and colleagues advocate a common-sense approach, elevating the importance of qualitative data, to ensure that decisions to intervene in humanitarian crises are timely and focused on reducing mortality (Robertson et al., 2002).

Conclusions

The specific challenges of monitoring and evaluating health interventions for conflict-affected populations require flexible and creative design, data collection and analysis. Conflict can severely disrupt health-system-generated data and require increased reliance on qualitative operational data. Monitoring and evaluation must consider beneficiary needs and perspectives, analyse context, and reference international conventions and standards to ensure applicability of results. The following chapter discusses security and protection issues.

Feedback on activities

Feedback on Activity 10.1

You could have focused on distribution of long-lasting insecticide-treated bednets (LLINs) through a public–private partnership, given the existence of untreated nets and an active private sector. In this case, your logframe may look somewhat like the one below:

Objectives	Indicators	Sources of Verification	Advocacy
Overall Reduce malaria mortality	By 15% from a baseline of 15.4/1,000 by the end of the 2yr project	Malaria survey	• Quality treatment available
Impact Reduced malaria infection rate	By 30% from baseline determined by survey/ health facility records	Pre/post-intervention malaria survey	• Quality diagnostics and treatment available

Output Distribution of 500,000 LLINs	100% coverage (minus % loss/destroyed) by the end of the project	End-of-project community survey	• Supply chain and transport functional
Outcome People are protected from malaria vectors at night	% nightly usage increased from baseline	Community social survey	• Ministry of Health and partners strengthen malaria diagnosis and treatment • Communities use LLINs appropriately
Input LLINs	500,000 within the first 6 months of project start	Procurement records	• Procurement and customs procedures navigable

11 Security and protection

Michiel Hofman

Overview

The aim of this chapter is to describe key issues in the protection of beneficiaries, security of health staff, and risk mitigation against assaults on health functions. Health workers and institutions have a specificity of purpose in conflict zones that allows them special legal protections not given other humanitarian workers and structures, but exposes them to risks requiring careful management. Concepts and case studies from the protection literature and operational experience are used.

Learning outcomes

After completing this chapter you should be able to:

- identify the main risks to beneficiary populations, legal obligations to non-combatants, and protection strategies in conflict zones
- describe risks to health staff, security strategies, and legal issues related to medical care in conflict-affected settings
- discuss assaults on health functions and common risk mitigation strategies to protect health functions and infrastructure in conflict zones

Protection of patients

For war victims, health most often means survival, which in turn depends on access to those essentials of life, which are food, water and medical care. In many cases this access is a challenge that people already have to meet every day in time of peace. In time of war, the lack of security and the political interests involved can suddenly make the search for the basic essentials vastly more complicated.

(Perrin, 1996)

Case studies

Provincial hospital, Lashkar Gah, Helmand Province, Afghanistan, May 2009. In the courtyard of the hospital compound, there is a lot of activity. A construction project is under way, conducted by a local company and supervised by representatives of the donor, the British Department for International Development (DFID). Eight heavily armed men provide protection for these British supervisors, inside a cordon of armoured vehicles with their diesel engines running. Inside the hospital, British army engineers are busy installing an oxygen distribution system for the building, guarded by their heavily armed and uniformed colleagues. Beside the hospital, trucks hired by UNICEF are offloading food for the feeding centre inside the hospital. The trucks are guarded by local Afghan police forces. All that is missing, in this very active provincial hospital, is patients. Other than a few destitute elderly, who seem to use the hospital as a shelter, the wards are empty. The absence of patients is quickly explained by people living around the hospital. They are afraid. The hospital is built on the riverside, and just across it a small forest is used by opposition troops to launch rocket and mortar attacks on government and army buildings in the city. The people believed, with so many soldiers inside the compound, it would be seen as an army base and attacked from across the river.

The first job, when Médecins Sans Frontières took over running the hospital, was to convince local police, the British army, and private security firms linked to DFID workers to stay away from the hospital. This meant abandoning a number of long-term infrastructure projects. However, this was the only secondary care facility for the entire region, and priority was given to immediate health needs. Six months later huge 'no-weapons' signs adorned the gates and walls of the compound, all soldiers and armed personnel were gone, and the hospital was full to its 120-bed capacity.

Mogadishu, Somalia, September 2011. The four corners of the measles and malnutrition hospital compound, run by Médecins Sans Frontières in the centre of the city, are marked by watchtowers and heavily armed men overlook the streets beyond. The walls have triple layers of barbed wire. The gates are equipped with metal detectors for visitors and patients alike. Inside, a further contingent of armed men patrol the perimeter. The hospital is full beyond its 120-bed capacity, with 150 patients. When asked, the patients say they feel safe in this hospital compound, because security is addressed.

These two examples describe measures taken in medical facilities to provide a sense of protection for its beneficiaries – patients and their families. The protection strategies chosen were very different, but outcomes were the same – a feeling of protection appropriate to the particular setting. In both cases, protective measures were implemented by the agency responsible for the health structure. The health care provider is responsible for providing protection for its patients and reminding other parties of their obligations in this area.

Who needs protection

Generally, for humanitarian and development assistance agencies, this is the most vulnerable groups – those who have suffered most. In conflict, the focus is on protecting civilians, as they are assumed to have no active part or voice in the conflict affecting them. However, for those providing health care in these environments, such simple distinctions are not possible. The right to appropriate medical care should be extended to all sick and wounded, including any combatants. International humanitarian law (IHL) is worded to ensure medical care extends to all, as sick and wounded combatants are defined as civilians as soon as they have a medical condition. This aspect, specific to medical relief programmes, complicates protection in health services as wounded soldiers admitted to health facilities may be targeted for violence.

What constitutes protection

Simple prevention from physical harm is not sufficient. An example of how this type of definition can be abused by authorities was seen during the 1996 conflict in Burundi. The predominantly Tutsi Burundian army forcibly emptied Hutu villages to concentrate the Hutu population in 'regroupment camps' – large locked compounds guarded by the army. The government defended this as protecting people from conflict violence. Indeed, it shielded people from direct physical harm but robbed them of all other freedom and dignity. Slim and Bonwick give a definition of protection that addresses its complexity as bringing together the priorities of safety, dignity and material needs and capturing the importance of a person's completeness as a human being as a combination of physical, emotional, social, cultural and spiritual attributes (Slim and Bonwick, 2005: 32).

Legal obligations

These elements of protection are enshrined in several legal obligations to authorities, usually, though not exclusively, country governments. In conflict, non-state actors (e.g. armed rebel groups, occupying armies, peace-keeping forces) are bound by the same legal obligations. The three most relevant are international humanitarian law, international human rights law, and international refugee law, which now includes protection of internally displaced persons. Most states are signatories to one or all of these, obliging them to actively safeguard the rights enshrined. Several 'mandated' organizations are tasked with monitoring compliance and reminding states and non-state actors of their obligations. These include the International Committee of the Red Cross (ICRC), the guardians of IHL, and specialist UN agencies (e.g. UNHCR for displaced populations, OHCHR for human rights, UNICEF for women and children's rights). The existence of specially-mandated agencies does not absolve humanitarian providers of responsibilities to maximize protection for their beneficiaries. Actual implementation still rests with health care providers.

Protection strategies

The right strategy is context-dependent. The most important aspect of any strategy is consultation with local beneficiaries. This is the only way to learn what they think they need protection from and what measures will help them feel secure. The DFID development workers missed this step in the Afghan hospital example. As they felt personally secure with their armed guards, they assumed patients would also. Health care providers should consider the following when developing protection strategies in conflict environments:

- A hospital or health centre must provide protection for its patients from physical violence.
- To feel protected, all patients need a sense of freedom and dignity (e.g. respecting cultural rules on separation of men and women can be key).
- Specific measures to protect patients who are former combatants from their former adversaries may be necessary.
- Measures to ensure free and impartial access to health facilities may be necessary, as limitations in freedom of movement are a key consequence of conflict.

/ **Activity 11.1**
11.1.1 What legal protections can beneficiaries expect?
11.1.2 What protection issue distinguishes medical care from other humanitarian relief in conflict-affected settings?

Security of health staff

Risks to health staff

One of the main reasons why health systems collapse in times of conflict is the difficulty of retaining qualified staff in insecure areas. Maps may show existing health structures, suggesting health care coverage. On closer examination, however, many have no or very few qualified staff as those who can have left for safer areas. Doctors usually have the resources to leave, and often do so in the early stages of conflict. Therefore, maintaining health services in conflict requires incentivizing health staff to remain, which largely depends on the kind of protection an agency can offer. Additionally, in areas where qualified staff are completely absent, running health services requires external health staff – usually expatriates – who require specific security strategies in hostile environments.

Security for aid workers in hostile environments is generally perceived to have deteriorated in the past decade. Anecdotal evidence suggests more humanitarian workers are killed, kidnapped or seriously injured, reducing the numbers of humanitarian projects conducted in highly volatile environments. This perception is nuanced by an exhaustive review of statistics behind security incidents that shows:

- in absolute numbers, more than a doubling of the number of serious incidents involving humanitarian staff between 1997 and 2009;
- in relative terms, accounting for the increased numbers of international humanitarian workers, this increase is only about 20%;
- increases mostly affect national staff, with larger increases in numbers of national staff affected as compared to expatriate staff;
- large increases in numbers of directly targeted, politically motivated attacks, now representing more than half of all incidents;
- 60% of all incidents occurred in three countries (Afghanistan, Somalia and Sudan);
- between 2006 and 2009, a 350% increase in the number of abductions, mainly affecting expatriate staff;
- road travel remains the single most dangerous part of any humanitarian operation (Stoddard et al., 2006, 2009b).

Security approaches

Ensuring security for humanitarian staff has relied on implementation of the *security triangle* (Figure 11.1), a combination of acceptance (e.g. notices, symbols, relationships), physical protection (e.g. walls, barbed wire), and deterrence (e.g. security cameras, armed guards).

Humanitarian agencies, especially NGOs, have traditionally emphasized *acceptance*, relying on good relations with local communities and authorities to ensure they will

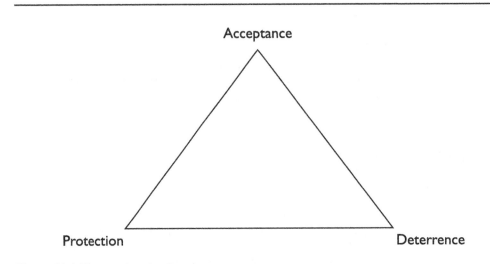

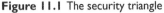

Figure 11.1 The security triangle

extend a measure of protection to the staff they host. Analysis of the past ten years shows this strategy is no longer effective in many conflicts, and agencies have begun adopting a range of protection and deterrence measures to ensure staff safety.

Stoddard and colleagues attribute the sharp increase in politically motivated and targeted attacks on humanitarian workers to the fact that, in the five countries with the highest number of incidents, humanitarian organizations are associated with government and occupying Western powers (Stoddard et al., 2009b). To reduce risks to staff, many agencies have implemented *negotiated access* to contact all armed groups, directly or indirectly, to convince them of the independence of the aid offered from political and military agendas. However, these investments seem to have had little effect on the number of targeted attacks on humanitarian workers.

With acceptance strategies failing, and little effect noted from the drive to change perceptions of collusion with Western powers (with the exception of the ICRC), the most common approaches organizations adopt to maximize staff security are as follows:

- *A very low profile.* For example, organizations do not put logos on buildings or cars, make little or no public announcement of organizational presence or activities, and allow only limited movement outside health facilities. The downside of this approach is that it nullifies any acceptance element, because if the organization is invisible to potential attackers, it is probably also invisible to local communities.
- *Strong deterrence.* This involves using armed protection for health structures and transport, including private security contractors. The downside of this approach is that in most contexts it militarizes the health facility, making it a target for attacks and endangering patients.
- *Delegation to national staff.* No longer posting expatriate staff in conflict zones to implement programmes, or subcontracting implementation to local NGOs, is often referred to as *remote management*. Objections to this approach include reduced accountability, reduced quality-assurance of projects, reduced impartiality, and increased pressure for diversion of resources. However, the biggest issue is the questionable ethics of *transfer of risk*.

Remote management is based on the premise that staff at greatest risk of involvement in security incidents should be removed, and expatriate staff are five times more likely to be involved in a serious security incident than national staff. The risk of kidnap contributes significantly to this statistic. The inconsistency in this reasoning is that expatriate and national staff are not actually exposed to the same risks, and Stoddard and colleagues argue that the nature of their work and local relationships mean national staff require specific security measures, proportionate to those for expatriate staff (Stoddard et al., 2009b). This can be illustrated by two specific risks: abduction and murder. Expatriates, especially Western expatriates, have the highest risk of abduction as the amount of ransom and political influence obtainable from their abduction is much greater. However, death threats to family members (e.g. to obtain agency resources) are highest for national staff, simply because the families of expatriates are not usually living in the conflict zone. It is impossible to quantify which of these risks is worse for victims, and remote management essentially transfers the risk of expatriate staff kidnapping to a risk of national staff or family murder.

Legal security for health staff

An additional risk, specific to humanitarian workers active in medical activities, is that of prosecution. This relates to the specific IHL requirement that health workers not distinguish between civilians and combatants. The risk of prosecution was demonstrated during the 2011 violence in Bahrain, when street protests in poor neighbourhoods of this Gulf state were forcibly repelled by government security forces with the help of the militaries of Saudi Arabia and the United Arab Emirates. The wounded, almost exclusively unarmed protesters, were treated in the central hospital. This was seen by authorities as a political act of health staff support of the uprising. Many doctors were consequently arrested, tried in military court, and given severe prison sentences in clear violation of IHL.

The *general protection of medical missions* is covered by IHL Article 16: Protocol I and Article 10: Protocol II. The latter states: 'Under no circumstances shall any person be punished for having carried out medical activities compatible with medical ethics, regardless of the person benefiting therefrom.' While these rules are not optional for signatory states to the Geneva Conventions, such as Bahrain, events in 2011 show this does not guarantee respect for medical staff immunity. So, in addition to strategies maximizing physical security for all staff, specific strategies to ensure legal security for health staff should be considered. While the ICRC can remind all authorities of these obligations, organizations are ultimately responsible for the security of their staff.

Activity 11.2

11.2.1 What risk to humanitarian staff has increased dramatically over the last 15 years, and how have humanitarian agencies responded?

11.2.2 Describe the most common strategies adopted when traditional 'acceptance' becomes ineffective.

11.2.3 Why are health staff exposed to specific legal risk when working in conflict zones?

Assaults on health functions

Case study

Afghanistan, 2009. This was a bad year for health care providers. A series of incidents highlighted the lack of respect among warring parties for the sanctity of health facilities. In May, a clinic in Khost province was destroyed and staff threatened by armed opposition fighters. In November, suspected militants burnt down a health clinic in the Daman district of southern Kandahar province. This was quickly condemned by Western forces as evidence that opposition groups, universally labelled *Taleban*, were indiscriminate in their violence. However, in late August Afghan and NATO forces had raided a clinic in Paktika province following reports of an opposition commander being treated inside. They killed 12 people with the support of helicopters firing at the building. One week later, US forces raided a hospital in Wardak province supported by the Swedish Committee for Afghanistan (SCA). Soldiers searched the hospital, forced bedridden patients out of rooms, and tied up staff and visitors. As they left, they ordered staff to report admissions of any suspected insurgents to coalition forces. These events suggest a complete disrespect for IHL by all parties in the conflict, as health structures are specifically protected from hostilities by the Geneva Conventions (e.g. Article 19ff/I, Article 22ff/II, Article 18ff/IV) and Articles 8ff/I and 7ff/II of the Additional Protocols. Article 11 of Protocol 11 stipulates:

1. *Medical units and transports shall be respected and protected at all times and shall not be the object of attack.*
2. *The protection to which medical units and transports are entitled shall not cease unless they are used to commit hostile acts, outside their humanitarian function. Protection may, however, cease only after a warning has been given, setting, whenever appropriate, a reasonable time-limit, and after such warning has remained unheeded.*

This may be the most important IHL section for all health care providers, as it means hospitals and health centres are seen as neutral space where patients can find relative safety within a conflict zone. The attacks on health facilities in Afghanistan in 2009 appear to breach this protection of medical missions, but closer examination shows the complexity of practical implementation of IHL in the field. The two incidents attributed to opposition forces were against facilities in which health care was either provided by the military, or military were protecting the NGO responsible for health care. Opposition forces regarded these health centres as military compounds, and attacked accordingly. Similarly, the attack by NATO did not occur in a vacuum. The USA and its allies have not recognized opposition troops as a legitimate army, but rather as terrorists to be treated as criminals. Local authorities, assisted by NATO, were thus entitled to enter health facilities to arrest criminals. Therefore, in both examples the warring party argued the IHL did not apply.

These arguments relate to a tricky aspect of IHL, which is the categorization of patients as former combatants or criminals. It is often wrongly assumed that patients, particularly those admitted to secondary care facilities, enjoy immunity from prosecution. In reality, each country has the right to enter a health facility with security forces (e.g. police, army, intelligence) to arrest or interrogate patients suspected of a crime. IHL only stipulates that a patient must be medically fit to be arrested or interrogated, or that the arresting party must provide access to similar medical treatment. IHL cannot stop police arresting a patient and transferring him or her to a prison hospital, but it does stipulate that the treating doctor must be consulted before security forces proceed. If similar medical treatment cannot be provided by arresting forces, this doctor can demand they wait until treatment is completed and the patient is declared medically fit.

Risk mitigation

Health structures cannot be assumed to provide safety on the basis of the IHL, which puts the onus on health care providers to actively ensure that health structures are as safe as possible. In most conflicts, this means ensuring that there can be no confusion about the function of the structure, and several measures can reduce misperceptions.

First, the presence of any military personnel in or around a medical structure is usually counter-productive as the structure will have the appearance of a military target. This precondition was absent in the health centre in Khost province, where the NGO chose to rely on NATO protection.

Second, a red cross, the internationally recognized sign for a medical facility should be displayed clearly on the walls and roof of the building, so its function is obvious and ground or aerial assaults reduced.

Third, clear negotiation with all warring parties is necessary to ensure all possible attackers are aware of the function of the building, and commit to respect IHL regarding the structure. As the Afghanistan case study shows, this cannot be assumed as both NATO and the Afghan army erroneously claimed exemptions from IHL because of the way they chose to classify opposition forces.

This classic approach is not possible in all contexts, and sometimes an alternative approach needs to be adopted like the non-aligned armed protection in the Somalia example or the low-profile approach in Afghanistan. The key lesson is that protection of health structures does not happen automatically. All strategies need active support by health care agencies to create a relatively safe environment for patients and staff. When implemented successfully, these strategies will transform a health facility into a physical manifestation of the often-quoted humanitarian space.

Activity 11.3

11.3.1 What steps need be taken to increase acceptance by warring parties of health structures as protected impartial zones?

11.3.2 What are the limitations of IHL in terms of protecting patients inside a health structure?

Conclusions

Providing health care in conflict zones has always been complex and potentially dangerous, but represents such an essential service that a level of risk seems justified. Worrying trends indicate less respect for the sanctity of medical missions as enshrined in the Geneva Conventions. Patients can no longer assume a health facility is a safe place, which puts the onus on medical providers to negotiate agreement with all warring parties that health structures are neutral physical manifestations of humanitarian space. Health staff face increased risk of targeted, political attacks, with acceptance strategies no longer mitigating risk. Acceptance remains the preferred security strategy in all contexts, including clear relationships with local communities and negotiated access with all armed groups. In contexts where acceptance has proved ineffective, alternative strategies include armed protection, low profile, or remote management. All have serious negative consequences and remain a last resort. IHL still provides the strongest legal protection health staff can use to protect patients, staff and structures. However, this is dependent on the willingness of nations, non-state actors, and multilateral forces to honour these laws. This requires ongoing negotiation and should not be assumed during conflict. The next section addresses transition, recovery, and strengthening health systems.

Feedback on activities

Feedback on Activity 11.1

11.1.1 The three most relevant international covenants giving a legal basis to protection are IHL (i.e. the Geneva Conventions) that ensures specific protection rights in conflict situations, international refugee law that ensures specific rights for refugees and displaced, and international human rights law that ensures individual rights in all situations.

11.1.2 International humanitarian law specifies that medical care in conflict situations is a guaranteed right for both civilians and combatants, defining a sick or wounded combatant, who has laid down his arms, as a de facto civilian.

Feedback on Activity 11.2

11.2.1 Since 1997, quantitative research shows a dramatic increase in the number of directly targeted, politically motivated attacks on humanitarian workers, as compared to the more circumstantial exposure to criminal attacks targeted at the resources relief operations represent.

11.2.2 When acceptance and negotiated access fail, humanitarian agencies increasingly revert to a low-profile (invisibility as a protection) approach, increased deterrence (armed protection) and delegation of implementation to national staff or national NGOs (remote management)

11.2.3 As health staff are obliged to treat all sick and wounded, including former combatants, this exposes them to the risk of prosecution by national security forces when combatants are from opposition parties.

Feedback on Activity 11.3

11.3.1 All parties in the conflict must be approached actively and agreements reached that particular structures are accepted as protected health facilities. Such an agreement usually requires the health structure to be demilitarized (i.e. a no-weapons policy implemented) and clearly marked with a red cross on the compound and roof to ensure that it cannot be mistaken for anything other than a health structure.

11.3.2 A country's official security forces (e.g. police, army, intelligence services) retain the right to enter health facilities and arrest or interrogate patients, when declared medically fit, or when equivalent medical service can be provided by security forces. In all cases, they cannot act without consultation with the doctor in charge of the patient.

SECTION III

Reconstruction

Transition and early recovery   12

Andre Griekspoor

Overview

The aim of this chapter is to describe the challenges of transition, including the links to early recovery and the necessity for humanitarian agencies to include an early recovery approach in their programmes. It is written primarily from the perspective of the international community engaged with crisis areas, supporting affected populations and their governments.

Learning outcomes

After completing this chapter you should be able to:

- identify key challenges and policy options for the health sector in transition, early recovery and recovery
- describe post-conflict needs assessment, recovery planning, and a common framework for analysing humanitarian, early recovery, and recovery needs
- discuss integrating early recovery and phasing-out strategies into humanitarian programmes

Transition and recovery challenges

When populations are affected by conflict, a first priority is providing humanitarian relief. For the health sector, this means reducing morbidity and mortality through essential health services guided by humanitarian principles. Rapid-impact humanitarian interventions need to focus on saving lives. However, equally necessary is strategic, medium- to long-term planning for health system recovery accounting for the pace of phasing-out relief activities.

In protracted crises, these development-oriented approaches may not be considered relevant until the conflict is clearly ending and a formal peace agreement process has started. Once formal recovery starts, the new government requests assistance of the main development partners (e.g. UN agencies, World Bank, European Union) with a *post-conflict needs assessment* to start planning for reconstruction and recovery.

Transition refers to the period when conflict appears to end, stabilization increases, and early government-led reconstruction and recovery efforts begin in partnership with the international community. Transition from acute or protracted conflicts incurs many challenges. Some humanitarian agencies have difficulties adapting to work that is no longer fully independent but aligned with national policies and in partnership with often weakened national health authorities. Transition phase funding is often complex, with humanitarian donors reducing their budgets, while development donors are still hesitant to begin. This may be because parts of the country are not yet fully secure, or because the conditions required for effective development (e.g. good governance, financial accountability) are not yet in place.

This negatively affects coverage and continuity of service delivery. For example, a 2006 evaluation in Liberia identified a major **transition funding gap** in the health sector, as humanitarian donors phased out, but development donors were not yet ready to step in. When confronted with the consequences of a fragmented and disrupted health system at the end of a long conflict, one cannot help asking why more was not done during the crisis to mitigate this. In South Sudan, current recovery faces severe shortages of all cadres of health workers. An almost total absence of education during three decades of war means it is now almost impossible to find people with sufficient secondary schooling to enrol in basic nursing and midwifery training, let alone medical education. Instead, cohorts of lower-cadre health workers are being trained by NGOs, each using their own curricula, with few leading to professional accreditation.

A key lesson is that recovery activities should not wait for formal, large-scale reconstruction and development programmes likely to be implemented in a later phase. Many interventions and approaches should begin during the humanitarian relief phase. The ideal of linking relief to recovery and development is seldom achieved, largely because the two approaches are separated by different instruments and processes. One way to create the necessary connection between relief and development is to use a common framework to identify humanitarian needs and opportunities for early recovery during crises, using the same health system logic as the basis for assessment and analysis for recovery.

Definitions and principles of transition

Transition is used here to describe the change from conflict to peace, and the subsequent shift between humanitarian and development programming. Transition is often associated with recovery, and overlaps with concepts such as early recovery, stabilization, and peace- and state-building. Most of these terms are ill-defined and interpreted differently by different stakeholders. Figure 12.1 shows these concepts in a spectrum between conflict and peace.

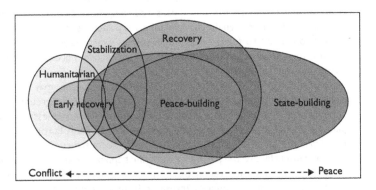

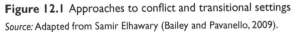

Figure 12.1 Approaches to conflict and transitional settings

Source: Adapted from Samir Elhaway (Bailey and Pavanello, 2009).

Transition is a complex non-linear process, with unclear beginnings, unpredictable outcomes, and high risks of falling back into a new conflict. It is often characterized by an uncertain period of 'no war, no peace', sometimes with dual administrations, coexistence of different geographical security situations, simultaneous humanitarian and recovery needs, and reduced humanitarian space. Part of the country may be stable with development programming, other parts may be in transition or still have humanitarian programming, as seen in DRC and Sudan. It is difficult to judge when transition and recovery start and when they end. Indications of the start of transition include declining levels of violence, improved security, decreasing levels of mortality and malnutrition, voluntary return of displaced populations, formal ceasefires and signing of peace agreements.

Transition and subsequent post-conflict recovery usually take much longer than expected when a peace agreement is signed and the first elected government takes office in transition. The 20 fastest-reforming countries in the twentieth century took 15–30 years, a generation, to raise institutional performance from very fragile to more resilient levels. It took an average 17 years to reduce military interference in politics, and 27 years to establish rules-based controls against corruption (World Bank, 2011).

The transition period signifies the following shifts in international engagement (OECD/INCAF, 2010):

- from humanitarian aid modalities, normally bypassing the state, to development aid that regards the state as primary partner and channel;
- from short-term focus on life-saving activities to a longer-term engagement aimed at establishing sustainable peace and viable state structures;
- from respecting humanitarian principles of humanity, impartiality and independence to aligning with peace-building and state-building objectives;
- from working with mainly international organizations to working with local partners.

Early recovery, recovery and development

Early recovery is the application of development principles to humanitarian situations, to stabilize national and sub-national capacities from further deterioration, so they can provide the foundation for full recovery and stimulate spontaneous recovery activities within affected populations (UNDP, 2008). Early recovery efforts need to begin in all sectors during initial relief efforts (e.g. during the acute emergency phase) so the necessary foundations for fully fledged recovery work are in place for the prolonged post-conflict transition or chronic emergency periods.

Recovery is the process of restoring the capacities of government and communities to rebuild and recover from crisis and preventing relapses. In so doing, recovery seeks not only to catalyse sustainable development activities but also to build upon earlier humanitarian programmes and ensure their inputs become assets for development (UNDP, 2001).

Development, in operational terms, describes operations that have long-term objectives, extending beyond two years, and presume conditions of security and a functioning administration pursuing national objectives and strategies in partnership with external actors (UNDP, 2001).

In this chapter, early recovery and recovery fall within the concept of transition. 'Early recovery' is defined as those interventions and approaches integrated within the humanitarian mandate. 'Recovery' is used here for those interventions and approaches that are part of formal post-conflict needs assessment and its recovery plan that connects directly with development mandates.

Rehabilitation, reconstruction and recovery

These terms are sometimes used to sequence phases or activities taking place following emergency response and relief activities. The terms overlap or can have very different temporalities in different contexts. Relief activities may continue for months or even years, while reconstruction may parallel ongoing relief activities, even within the same population groups and areas (Lavell, 2000).

Rehabilitation and reconstruction do not have agreed definitions. Rehabilitation overlaps with humanitarian interventions and generally refers to initial, often temporary, re-establishment of infrastructure and functionality to meet the needs of local economic and welfare requirements.

Reconstruction often describes more permanent physical reconstruction of damaged infrastructure and replacement of assets to pre-disaster levels. This may include rebuilding so that the infrastructure is more resilient to future hazards (e.g. adherence to earthquake-resistant building codes). Recovery generally includes the notion of 'building back better' and planning for disaster risk reduction. It may encompass all infrastructure aspects, but certainly includes restoration and improvement of livelihoods and living conditions of conflict-affected communities. (UNISDR, 2009).

Humanitarian versus development aid

Many donor countries separate their development and humanitarian funding, with related information split accordingly. Both have distinctly different procedures and planning frameworks. Table 12.1 describes typical dimensions of humanitarian versus development aid. Given these differences, it is clearer why the transformation from humanitarian to development aid cannot be linear. Transition requires both types of aid in parallel.

Activity 12.1

Identify important international and national actors and the roles they could play in early recovery of the health sector.

Assessment and planning

Post-conflict needs assessment and recovery planning

Needs during and after crises are enormous, particularly in fragile and low- to low-middle-income countries, and invariably disproportionate to the capacities of

Table 12.1 Differences in humanitarian and development aid architecture

	Humanitarian	Development
Guiding principles	Good Humanitarian Donorship	Paris Declaration, Accra, Fragile States Principles, the High Level Forum Busan 'new deal'
Overall lead	OCHA	Government and lead donors
Coordination structure	IASC cluster approach	Sector-wide approach, International Health Partnership
Sector or cluster working groups	Education, WASH, food security, health, early recovery, etc.	Education, infrastructure, agriculture and livelihoods, health, public finance, etc.
Needs identification	Humanitarian Assessments	Post-conflict needs assessment
Prioritized plans	Common Humanitarian Action Plan, consolidated appeals process	National development plan, Country Assistance Framework, Poverty Reduction Strategy Paper, bilateral plans, Transitional Results Framework
Funds	Central Emergency Response Fund, common humanitarian funds bilateral funds	Peace-building funds, multi-partner trust funds, bilateral funds, international financial institutions
Actors	Government agencies, UN agencies, international NGOs, humanitarian donor sections	Government agencies, bilateral development donor sections, World Bank, UN agencies, NGOs, civil society organizations

Source: OECD/INCAF (2010).

international community and national governments to fund and implement necessary interventions. Prioritization becomes a difficult technical process, often politically charged and requiring complex compromises among different actors. A joint declaration by the European Commission (EC), United Nations Development Group (UNDG) and the World Bank has agreed to assist crisis-affected countries in reconstruction and recovery planning (EC et al., 2008). *Post-conflict needs assessment* (PCNA) was conceived in the early 2000s to address these challenges through multi-sectoral, multi-stakeholder approaches and short to medium time-frames. It requires a complex analytical process led by national authorities, supported by the international community, and conducted by multilateral agencies collaborating with national and civil society stakeholders (UNDP et al., 2004). PCNAs aim to overcome consequences of conflict, prevent renewed outbreaks, shape short- and potentially mid-term recovery priorities, and articulate financial implications based on an overall long-term vision.

Post-conflict needs assessment methods

PCNA differs from post-disaster needs assessment (PDNA) because of the need to address the complexities of conflict. PDNAs are guided by a specific handbook and damage and loss assessment methods (ECLAC, 2003). PCNAs are guided by the *Practical Guide to Multilateral Needs Assessments in Post-conflict Situations* (UNDP et al.,

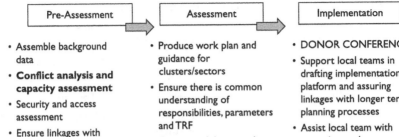

Figure 12.2 The post-conflict needs assessment (PCNA) process
Source: Yao (2004).

2004), conflict analysis (http://pcna.undg.org/) and capacity assessment tools (UNDG, 2009), and the Transitional Result Framework (TRF) and Matrices (TRM) have been put forward for reporting (UNDG, 2008). As shown in Figure 12.2, PCNAs have three phases: (i) pre-assessment, (ii) assessment, and (iii) implementation.

Post-conflict needs assessment challenges

Methodological challenges, particularly in developing the recovery plan, include:

- costing PCNA recovery plans, including allocation of funding needs between sectors and predicting future funding needs;
- opportunity costs of the PCNA, as it can sometimes take over a year with significant inputs from all stakeholders;
- risks of recreating the same political and social structures at the root of the conflict, given the political nature of the PCNA process;
- when national policy-making capacity is still weak, dominant international agencies, donors and experts are often free to push politically oriented policy options rather than understanding what is best for each context;
- time-frames are limited and often unrealistic, reducing consultation with all stakeholders;
- technical excellence is difficult when using the unreliable, incomplete information found in fragile settings;
- assessments and recovery planning done in isolation will be insufficiently embedded into either humanitarian coordination or longer-term development cooperation mechanisms.

Health system analysis for recovery planning

A lesson learned from post-conflict recovery planning is to invest early in systematic analysis of the health sector. This should start in the early phases of crises, and be elaborated as the crisis progresses, so that much of the pre-assessment work will have been completed before the formal PCNA starts. Thus, initial ideas for post-conflict recovery and policies will have been formulated (Pavignani and Colombo, 2009: Module 13). No single method is applicable to all data analysis for the health sector. Multiple sources of primary and secondary data, pre- and post-crisis, are necessary and often require different data collection methods. Methods include *health facility-based surveys*, assessing damage and functionality using the health cluster *Health Resource Availability Mapping* tool, qualitative capacity assessment of provincial and district health authorities, workshops with ministry of health departments, document reviews, and semi-structured interviews with humanitarian providers (e.g. NGOs, UN agencies, donors). To ensure analytical consistency, the WHO health system framework, with its six health system building blocks (Figure 12.3), can be used as a common guide for early recovery and recovery needs assessments.

Under service delivery, the first building block, WHO lists seven subsectors that should provide essential programmes throughout relief and recovery phases then expand to more comprehensive services:

- general clinical services
- child health
- nutrition
- infectious diseases
- sexual and reproductive health
- non-infectious diseases, including injuries and mental health
- environmental health.

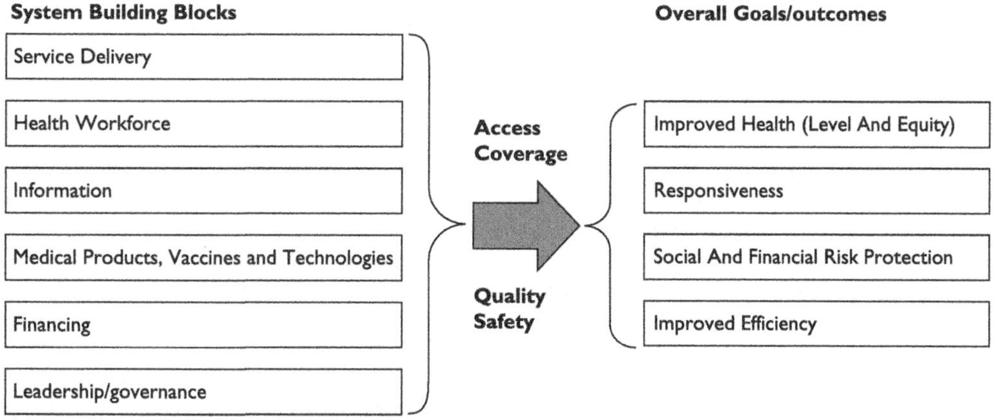

Figure 12.3 WHO health system framework
Source: WHO (2007b).

The five steps for health sector analysis, including the essential health programmes, are as follows:

1. *Determine pre-conflict baseline*: health status and pre-existing health risks, perform-ance of health programmes and the health system, existing policies, health system preparedness (e.g. strategies, action plans, disaster risk management).
2. *Estimate the impact of conflict*: on disease burden, health infrastructure and function-ality (e.g. service delivery), impacts averted by prevention and mitigation efforts, health system response capacity.
3. *Response*: includes humanitarian and early recovery interventions to address changes in the disease burden, re-establishing life-saving services, restoring health system functionality.
4. *Recovery strategy*: planning for outcomes, outputs, and monitoring indicators with short- and medium-term targets (e.g. integrating disaster and emergency risk management into health strategy and preparedness planning).
5. *Estimate costs*: to address reconstruction and recovery needs based on *building back better* approaches.

Analytical framework for humanitarian response, early recovery and recovery

We propose an analytical framework, incorporating the elements above, to identify health recovery priorities (Table 12.2). This matrix, adapted from the health components of PDNA, can serve as a standardized protocol, with reference indicators added to guide systematic data collection and provide examples of recovery interventions.

Opportunities and options for post-conflict health sector recovery

The post-conflict recovery period is often characterized by enthusiasm and renewed energy. Once elected, the new government often wants to deliver on the peace divi-dend and reform the systems in place before or during conflict, to break with the past and move into the future. This pressure for change and modernization, along with favourable international relationships and potentially expanded funding, can reduce the normal opposition to reforms.

Policy-makers with resource constraints face the strategic dilemma of prioritizing the scale-up of a limited set of health interventions to the entire population or strengthening key health system components and progressively expanding comprehen-sive primary care district by district. Rapid scale-up approaches may temporarily exclude equity, favouring coverage of as many people as possible, as quickly and cheaply as possible. Hard-to-reach populations (e.g. geographically, economically, socially) are the last to benefit from rapid scaling up, unless deliberate efforts are made to include them. Extra efforts may be justified on epidemiological (e.g. hard-to-reach groups are high-risk) or fairness grounds (e.g. when hard-to-reach groups have been deliberately excluded before or during conflict). However, equity concerns should not lead to 'lowest common denominator' approaches of equal access for all to poor-quality services.

Table 12.2 Analytical framework for health sector recovery

Health programmes and health system functions	Pre-crisis challenges and distortions in baseline health sector indicators	Impact of conflict, further challenges and distortions for early recovery	Humanitarian response	Early recovery options	Recovery options
1a. Service (programme) delivery					
– general clinical services					
– child health					
– nutrition					
– infectious diseases					
– sexual and reproductive health					
– non-infectious diseases					
– environmental health					
1b. Service delivery, organization and management (e.g. health network infrastructure, equipment, transport)					
2. Human resources for health					
3. Health information system					
4. Medical products, vaccines, technologies					
5. Health financing					
6. Leadership and governance					

Source: Adapted from WHO/HAC (2010).

Principles guiding the recovery process

The first principle guiding the recovery process is *early investment in systemic analysis of the health sector.* Work on health sector recovery should precede political developments. Health systems emerging from conflict are fragile, and adoption of blueprint models or quick fixes is far less effective than advocating for incremental changes. The initial focus should be on repair and getting things working, rather than reform.

The second principle is that *recovery should not aim to restore the pre-conflict health system*. Changes will have occurred, especially during protracted crises, providing opportunities to redress some of the problems affecting the original system. Only comprehensive analysis can detect these opportunities, enabling advocacy for appropriate remedies. Table 12.3 provides examples of possible policy responses to common challenges.

Table 12.3 Key health system challenges and response options

Common flaws and key challenges	Possible policy responses	Examples and remarks
Leadership and governance		
Fragmented, inconclusive, evidence-free policy formulation	Establish or strengthen autonomous policy intelligence units and resource centres.	Disseminating reliable and relevant information is as important as producing it.
	Establish effective coordination venues.	The commitment of participants is stronger when the discussion is centred around concrete operational issues.
	Promote wide, evidence-based policy discussion.	Difficult to put into practice for weak and often contested governments, constrained by limited capacity and inadequate information, and under pressure with daily operations.
	Introduce aid management instruments that force participants to agree shared policies.	'Shadow' aligning donor interventions is an obvious strategy for fragmented health systems, where weak health authorities are unable to play a leading role. Always very labour-intensive and often controversial.
Ineffective management systems	Introduce competitive, fixed-term appointment schemes for management positions.	Imply a break with traditional civil service provisions. Easier to establish within a contracting-out framework.
	Introduce performance-related rewards and sanctions for managers.	
	Encourage the emergence of professional managers.	Always difficult in health sectors dominated by medical doctors. A sizeable investment in the training of professional managers must be complemented by provisions aimed at strengthening management practice.
	Reduce civil service constraints and controls.	Easier to achieve after the collapse of state functions.
	Decentralize accountability.	A weak central government is often at pains to keep together a fractured country, as in Afghanistan. Decentralization in these cases is praised in the policy discourse, but hardly pursued in practice.
	Introduce transparent and regular external audits, carried out according to international standards.	Although constant sources of controversy, formal external audits are valuable to control abuses, as well as to foster the emergence of indigenous capacity. Effective audits demand high technical capacity, not always granted.
	Solve conflicts of interests.	

Health workforce

Bloated, under-skilled workforce	Freeze recruitment of unskilled and low-skilled staff.	Politically difficult to enforce, particularly in decentralized settings. The peace process (as in Angola) may imply the incorporation of rebel health workers into the workforce, in this way further expanding its ranks.
	Expand training of high-skilled cadres.	The lack of educated candidates to enrol into health courses may undermine this approach. Also, recruiting indigenous and appropriate skilled trainers is usually difficult. Unrealistic training plans are commonplace in recovery processes.
	Retrain/upgrade existing staff.	Special challenges are provided by the proliferation of volunteer or semi-volunteer health workers, common in contexts dominated by NGOs, as in Afghanistan or Southern Sudan. A long-term accreditation programme is needed to professionalize these cadres.
	Introduce incentives to promote retrenchment.	Unaffordable for many resource-starved health sectors. Given the unemployment prevalent in many distressed contexts, retrenchment may represent a politically unacceptable option. Well-designed incentive packages are needed to retain competent cadres, while ballast workers are encouraged to leave. Always difficult to achieve.
Rigid civil service regulations, resulting in inefficient and unresponsive workforce	Introduce fixed-term, performance-based contracts.	It can be introduced as an interim measure to fill hardship positions, often with NGOs as sub-contractors. Later, it can be expanded to affect larger parts of the workforce.
	Devolve hiring and firing responsibilities to local health authorities directly involved in health care provision.	Demands fairly robust management capacity at local level. Fungible budget provisions may encourage efficient allocations.

Medical products and technologies

Overpriced and scarce drugs	Establish a centralized purchasing system of generic drugs through international competitive bidding.	The purchasing system may be operated by government authorities or by non-profit organizations. A weak MoH might prefer to delegate drug supply duties to external agencies. Inappropriate donor requirements may impede their participation into efficient procurement schemes.
	Standardize treatment protocols.	
	Promote the essential drug concept.	

(Continued overleaf)

Table 12.3 Continued

Common flaws and key challenges	Possible policy responses	Examples and remarks
Health financing		
Insufficient financing, absolute or against stated goals	Narrow the scope of health service provision.	Politically very difficult. No known examples of explicit policies in this sense. Often carried out quietly, in an escapist way, generally with unsatisfactory results.
	Advocate for additional funding (internal and external). Negotiate loans with development banks.	Poor absorption may reduce the benefits of expanded financing. A convincing cost analysis may help raise additional funding.
	Capture existing financing, such as informal charges.	May yield substantial returns in middle-income settings. In very poor ones, service delivery must remain heavily subsidized (explicitly or not).
High operational costs, due to the dispersion of tasks and activities	Correct existing inefficiencies in service provision.	Often neglected, both in practice and in the policy discourse, usually emphasizing the need for additional resources.
	Encourage the merging of some functions, like drug supply, training, data collection.	Easier to achieve if linked to convincing policies and realistic goals.
Service delivery		
Large portions of the population without access to basic services	Invest in underserved areas.	Mozambique in 1990s. Usually depending on donor largesse. If not well planned and managed, it can create or reinforce serious distortions.
	Design and introduce low-cost service delivery packages.	Service delivery in underserved areas lacking basic infrastructures is usually more expensive than anticipated.
	Introduce incentives to encourage staff redeployment.	Mozambique in 1990s. Staff housing was included in rehabilitated or new facilities, drug supply to peripheral facilities was granted.
	Offer incentives to promote exemption schemes for the poor.	Difficult to achieve.
	Remove or reduce formal and informal user charges.	Informal charges may be stopped only by adequately financing health service provision.
	Launch community health worker programmes.	Difficult to sustain and to expand. Of limited effectiveness without the support of performing formal health services.
Unbalanced, derelict network	Develop cost-effective functional categories of health facilities.	
	Allocate investments to cover neglected areas and populations.	Mozambique in 1990s.
	Develop cost-effective functional categories of health facilities.	

Hospital-oriented sector	Close down some redundant and derelict hospitals.	Always highly contentious. Attempts are under way in Kosovo.
	Downsize some hospitals, while rehabilitating them.	
	Build new first-referral hospitals in areas deprived of them.	Mozambique in 1990s.
	Design primary health care-oriented training programmes.	Mozambique in 1990s.
Deregulated privatization of service provision	Contract out service delivery (e.g. NGOs, charities).	Cambodia in 1990s.
	Contract out regulatory functions and/or other services. Increase salaries.	Mozambique in the 1990s and recently Angola. Insufficient to curb widespread practice, if not associated with complementing regulatory measures.
	Regulate payments	Difficult to achieve when the practice has become entrenched.

Source: Pavignani and Colombo (2009: Module 12).

Activity 12.2

Choose a post-conflict country with which you are familiar and, using Figure 12.3 and Table 12.2 consider which of the six WHO building blocks you might address first to strengthen the health system.

Early recovery and phasing out humanitarian programmes

Early recovery

The general consensus is that early recovery should be integrated into humanitarian responses as soon as possible. Recent humanitarian reform through the cluster system aims to improve the 'predictability, timeliness and effectiveness of humanitarian response and pave the way for recovery'. This resonates with humanitarian evaluation criteria of connectedness, to look at whether activities of a short-term emergency nature were conducted in a way that took longer-term problems into account (Hallam, 1998). However, the literature is not clear on what humanitarian agencies can do to strengthen early recovery, as a precise distinction between humanitarian and early recovery interventions is rarely possible. Donors could provide clarity on what to include as early recovery in humanitarian proposals, as Good Humanitarian Donorship Principle 9 references support for linking relief to recovery. Several principles can guide the transition to early recovery:

- Do not undermine national systems.
- Work with national health authorities and partners where possible, and develop national capacity when possible.

- Establish the foundation for coherent health system functions as part of humanitarian approaches.
- Use the health system analysis framework to identify priorities and opportunities for early recovery, and connect with longer-term recovery and health system reforms.
- Create an environment in which development partners can connect early.

The health cluster is not well-prepared to manage early recovery. As its mandate is emergency response, expertise in early recovery analysis is often lacking. The health system building blocks provide practical examples of ways the humanitarian community can support early recovery.

Governance and service delivery

This is usually compromised during conflict. Early recovery approaches aim to connect with national and sub-national health authorities in overall coordination of the health sector. As outlined in the 2011 *IASC Guidance Note on Working with National Authorities*, clusters should support or complement existing national response and preparedness coordination mechanisms wherever possible (IASC, 2011b). Where appropriate, and as early as possible, government or suitable national counterparts should co-chair cluster meetings with the cluster lead agency.

In practice, the cluster approach may not be familiar to national health authorities. A briefing package, and regular updates on the health cluster and what can be expected from it, will help address such lack of familiarity. At national levels, MoH is often represented at cluster meetings in a role of low responsibility, and as such may send junior technical staff. At peripheral levels, the situation may be less politically complex, with provincial health authorities chairing or co-chairing cluster meetings. International agencies can maintain separate meetings to discuss sensitive issues if partners consider that national authorities are not respecting humanitarian principles.

Depending on changing contexts, national health authorities should start chairing health sector meetings. Where appropriate, international humanitarian agencies can build management capacity among sub-national health authorities (e.g. by supporting joint supervision visits to health facilities). It is likely that preparedness activities will be an increasing portion of the work. Cluster lead agencies and partners should ensure that, during crises, their coordination mechanisms and activities support national emergency preparedness efforts. During transition, efforts and resources should be directed towards ensuring national response mechanisms are equipped for better mitigating the effects of future crises. In the health sector, this often means establishing disease early warning surveillance systems.

Humanitarian coordination meetings should connect with development coordination, for example by organizing joint technical meetings on issues of common concern. Health cluster partners should be invited to PCNA processes. NGOs with a dual humanitarian and transition mandate and national NGOs can participate in health coordination meetings.

Health cluster partners are often unaware of national policies and guidelines. These should be updated as necessary in close collaboration with the national health authorities. The health cluster can facilitate standardization of agreements between health authorities and cluster partners on essential service packages, performance-related incentives for health care staff, and joint supervision and training. For example, instead of establishing temporary health units, agencies can strengthen an existing nearby health facility.

Human resources

In protracted conflicts, humanitarian agencies often invest in creating cadres of community health workers through ad hoc agency-specific courses. This can create expectations that these cadres will be integrated into the health system workforce post-crisis, when the new ministry of health does not actually have the resources to do so. Higher salaries or incentives paid by humanitarian agencies may drain staff from the national health system. Agency **human resources development** and management should minimally avoid further undermining development of the future health sector workforce, and collaborate during recovery. For example, agencies can work with national health authorities to develop consistent standards, training curricula, post descriptions, remuneration packages and a national human resources for health database.

Pharmaceuticals

Humanitarian agencies often have specific procurement channels for pharmaceuticals. Orders are often placed with international suppliers, as they are more competitive and can provide better quality assurance. Consequently, national supply channels may break down. Agencies should minimally avoid further undermining national capacities and support recovery by agreeing an essential medicines list. Additionally, health cluster partners can seek to certify pharmaceutical quality, including that of local providers. Central procurement centres can sometimes be established on behalf of humanitarian agencies. These can later be handed over to government or privatized through a national NGO.

Health information systems

Multiple information systems may be created, undermining the functioning of a uniform national health management information system (HMIS). To support recovery, consensus on standardized surveillance and health facility reporting forms can be sought. HMIS functionality in sub-national health offices should be created or strengthened, starting minimally with early warning systems (e.g. EWARN). To promote HMIS usage, service delivery incentives can be linked to complete and accurate reporting. Humanitarian agencies can assist sub-national health offices with analysis, dissemination and decision-making.

Health financing

The way health services are financed affects the quality and accessibility of services significantly (WHO, 2010c). Debates on maintaining or introducing user fees focus on supporting sustainable health financing rather than the right to health and humanitarian principles (e.g. that humanitarian interventions should be provided according to need, accessible without discrimination, and affordable to all). In principle, humanitarian health services should be provided free at the point of delivery (IASC, 2010b). Before deciding to abolish or maintain user fees during transition, policy-makers should examine the impact of existing regulations and practices on health services access and their influence on equity, usage, and quality of care. Humanitarian and government stakeholders should be involved policy discussions about developing equitable financing mechanisms.

Phasing out humanitarian coordination mechanisms

Planning humanitarian exit strategies as needs decrease should be an integral part of overall strategy planning among agencies. If possible, agencies should work closely with national authorities from the beginning on transition planning. Many international agencies have dual humanitarian and development mandates, and are likely to continue their support beyond addressing humanitarian needs and early recovery. Such agencies will need to engage with health development coordination, led by the national health authorities, in addition to humanitarian coordination.

The process of deactivation and phasing out is not as simple as activation. There is no defined moment in time when the humanitarian phase ends. Pre-conflict health system distortions, marginalization of vulnerable groups and access inequities may still exist, while remaining pockets of humanitarian need and risks of conflict relapse may justify continued humanitarian intervention. As mortality and malnutrition rates fall below emergency thresholds, the situation needs to be interpreted carefully as stopping humanitarian interventions could lead to these rates increasing.

The decision to deactivate humanitarian response mechanisms should always include a risk assessment and conflict analysis. Phasing out is a negotiated process with no single reference for the decision. The capacity of the affected government to manage residual consequences of the conflict requires consideration. The government may declare the crisis over at some point, which deactivates the cluster mechanism, though it may be replaced by a recovery coordination mechanism (e.g. Pakistan). The capacity of development partners to support longer-term recovery should also be considered. In practice, capacity limitations of humanitarian agencies and declining donor interest will also determine deactivation. Three options for deactivating humanitarian coordination are as follows:

1. *Closing the humanitarian coordination mechanism.* This can be done by government initiative, due to political interest in bringing a close to the humanitarian phase, or by the international community deciding the humanitarian mandate is no longer required.
2. *Shifting coordination leadership from humanitarian the international community to national health authorities.* This requires in-depth capacity assessment and possibly interventions to strengthen capacity (Potter and Brough, 2004).
3. *Transforming humanitarian coordination into disaster risk management.* This requires creating or strengthening a risk management unit within the ministry of health, and applies more to post-disaster than post-conflict contexts.

Conclusions

This chapter introduces concepts related to transition and early health system recovery. Recovery requires in-depth analysis of the health system, existing strengths and weaknesses, and how it was affected by conflict. The key approach for both transition and early recovery is shifting from short-term life-saving to longer-term engagement with the state as primary partner. The next chapter discusses health system strengthening in greater detail.

Feedback on activities

Feedback on Activity 12.1

Some of the actors and activities you may have included are outlined below, but this list is not intended to be exhaustive:

Actors	Potential roles
National government	• co-leadership of transition and recovery • mobilization of donor resources • strategy development and mechanisms for health service delivery (e.g. agreeing minimum service package) • coordinating development of essential drugs list • establishing a central pharmaceutical depot • recruiting doctors and public health staff • coordinating development and maintenance of HMIS • coordinating delivery of health services
UN agencies	• technical support in all the above, depending on individual mandates and interests
NGOs/private sector	• staffing and provision of medical services • supporting functioning health facilities • organizations with their own sources of income can provide human, financial and material resources (e.g. consultants, staff salaries, training, essential supplies) • input into policy formulation if appropriate
Donors	• funds to support services, vertical programmes, or reference hospitals • funds for training essential human resources (e.g. nurses, midwives) • some provide funds for health sector staff salaries • subsidies or funds for essential drugs and supplies • support for specific health sector surveys and evaluations
Civil society	• develops functioning community health committees, to plan and oversee local health service provision • helps identify volunteer health workers • works with sub-national health authorities to ensure good health services

Feedback on Activity 12.2

While there may be examples of countries going through a post-conflict transition in which one or two blocks are addressed first, in reality all building blocks should be tackled simultaneously. They overlap, and trying to preferentially address one or more can contribute to ineffective health system strengthening.

Post-conflict health system strengthening

Annemarie ter Veen and Steve Commins

Overview

The aim of this chapter is to describe key concepts in health system strengthening in fragile and post-conflict settings. It expands on concepts of transition, recovery, and health system building blocks from the previous chapter.

Learning outcomes

After completing this chapter, you should be able to:

- identify responses and actors in post-conflict health system strengthening
- describe key aspects of post-conflict health system reconstruction in relation to the six health system building blocks
- consider monitoring and evaluation of health system strengthening initiatives

Health system strengthening responses: the post-conflict transition

The moment a state becomes 'post-conflict' can be defined by the signing of a formal peace agreement (i.e. military transition), a political transition by elections, or a negotiated or military power transfer, and the perception among national and international actors of an opportunity for peace and recovery.

Humanitarian responses are the primary means of health sector support in contexts of deteriorating governance, arrested development, and the early stages of post-conflict transition. As government may lack capacity and resources to ensure public services are delivered, humanitarian agencies fill the gaps. The post-conflict period, the primary focus of this chapter, is an important time to rebuild lives and social systems, including the health system. Post-conflict transition is characterized by shifting emphasis from saving lives (i.e. humanitarian approach) to restoring livelihoods, achieving internationally agreed development goals, and increasing reliance on national ownership through national strategies (i.e. development approach).

Health system strengthening is a focus of development actors early on in the post-conflict transition process. Once some measure of peace and stability has been established, the focus shifts towards long-term processes. Figure 13.1 illustrates the transition from private and humanitarian health services during conflict to increasingly government-led service delivery post-conflict.

The transition from humanitarian relief to the early stages of development is complex and non-linear. While there is no 'one size fits all' approach to post-conflict health

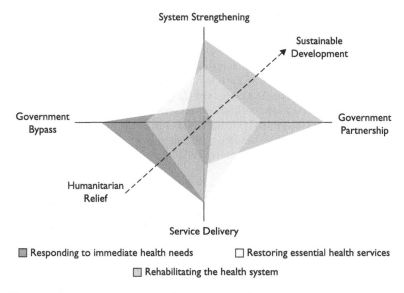

System Strengthening

Sustainable Development

Government Bypass — Government Partnership

Humanitarian Relief

Service Delivery

■ Responding to immediate health needs   □ Restoring essential health services
□ Rehabilitating the health system

Figure 13.1 Transitions to sustainable health system development
Source: Brinkerhoff (2008).

system strengthening; lessons can be learned from the approaches developed by various actors in other post-conflict settings. Chapter 12 introduced the six *WHO health system building blocks* as a framework for analysis and recovery planning. These building blocks encompass essential health system functions, and the model is applicable across the continuum from humanitarian relief to sustainable development.

Defining health system strengthening

WHO defines health system strengthening as building capacity in critical components of health systems to achieve more equitable and sustained improvements across health services and health outcomes, with health systems defined as the sum of all organizations, institutions, resources and people whose primary purpose it is to improve health (WHO, 2007b). Health system strengthening therefore requires a comprehensive approach addressing all components and collaboration of key actors within the health system.

Actors in health system strengthening

Successful health system strengthening requires engagement from key groups of actors who are generally different from those described in previous chapters. The gradual shift from humanitarian to development approaches triggers different support mechanisms within the international community (e.g. the development versus humanitarian system). National authorities, private sector and civil society will also need to adapt to this changing context.

Government. The health sector is the responsibility of the national and sub-national government. Health system strengthening can be a multi-level process, depending on the degree of decentralization in the health sector. The national ministry of health (MoH) is responsible for developing, implementing and monitoring national health policies, standards and regulations, coordinating all activities related to the health sector, and linking regional, local, and in some cases private health programmes with funding resources. The MoH must plan priorities based on the disease burden and available human, material and financial resources. Due to the influence of the Millennium Development Goals (MDGs), national health strategies in post-conflict countries often focus on poor communities equity (MDG1), child health (MDG4), maternal health (MDG5), infectious disease control (MDG6), and elements of gender (MDG3) and global partnerships (MDG8).

Donors. Most development donors also focus on MDG priorities, particularly in fragile states that are likely to prevent global achievement of the MDGs in 2015. Donors play a key role in supporting health service delivery and health system strengthening in post-conflict states, due to the influence they can leverage by setting funding priorities and conditions, which determines the direction of these processes. Their actions can sometimes weaken collaborative or coherent approaches to health system strengthening, as the structures and regulations of differing donor programmes being implemented can affect the relationships between MoH, other government agencies, service providers, local communities, and donors themselves. Alternatively, aid programmes can strengthen the role of government in health and improve its relationship with beneficiaries if they are well-planned and coordinated well. Planning and coordinating are major challenges in post-conflict reconstruction.

Considerable funding in conflict-affected and early post-conflict fragile states is delivered through short-term uncoordinated projects, rather than as part of a broader development strategy, because it avoids significantly weakened state structures. However, this fails to strengthen state systems or provide predictable and long-term funding, and improving aid delivery to post-conflict states is now firmly on donor agendas (OECD/DAC, 2007; GHD, 2003). There are inherent trade-offs between long-term state capacity-building and the **humanitarian imperative** to deliver services quickly. As crisis is ameliorated, donors wrestle with how to reduce the need for external aid and service providers and building internal service-delivery capacity without creating undue hardship for affected populations.

Non-state providers. These include large and small international and local NGOs, bilateral organizations, national development cooperation, faith-based organizations (FBOs), consultancy agencies, and academic institutions conducting capacity-building and research. They can be numerous, especially in post-conflict settings where donor interest and funding is abundant. Humanitarian non-state providers (NSPs) are accustomed to working in insecure environments and can often provide services where others cannot. However, the humanitarian assistance approach is less effective in laying the foundations for longer-term development and many humanitarian NSPs will leave as humanitarian funding is reduced. Other humanitarian NSPs are reluctant to work with national governments or certain international donors, instead working at community level to ensure they can provide services in an impartial and independent manner. Consultancy groups can leverage significant budgets and often work directly with health ministries during post-conflict recovery. They may also support contracting out of health services provision to NGOs and FBOs.

UN agencies. The UN system plays a major role in the health sector. The main UN health actors (i.e. WHO, UNICEF, UNFPA, the World Bank) are collectively known as

H4, although with the recent addition of UNAIDS there are now five agencies. WHO generally offers technical support in health system strengthening, human resources, **disease surveillance**, and disease control. Part of UNICEF's mandate is child health, and it focuses on activities such as training health staff in the integrated management of childhood illnesses and vaccine supply for the expanded programme on immunization. UNFPA focuses on reproductive health and large demographic surveys (e.g. national census). The World Bank is a major development donor. UNAIDS provides technical and material support for HIV and AIDS prevention and control. During the later stages of post-conflict recovery, the focus of activity within the UN agencies gradually shifts from sections focusing on humanitarian assistance to those with a clearer mandate to support health systems strengthening.

Civil society. Communities play a vital role in post-conflict development. In humanitarian contexts, when state fragility is at its greatest, communities may need to ensure their own health, welfare, and survival. However, without external support these efforts are seldom sustainable. During active conflict, community support structures may be dysfunctional due to insecurity or displacement. Once functional health facilities are in place, generally due to public or NSP support, communities and existing civil society organizations may choose to participate in local health governance structures (e.g. Community Health and Development Committees in DRC). Often these committees are initially concerned with establishing community-based services through recruiting volunteer health workers. It is not until a more stable situation develops that committees begin monitoring and evaluating service quality.

Activity 13.1

Consider one or more post-conflict countries in which you are interested.

13.2.2 Do you think that the length of time during which there was a lack of proper governance has had an effect on the severity of disruption of the health system?

13.2.3 What other factors could play a role?

Key aspects of health system strengthening

None of the six **health system strengthening building blocks** represents a stand-alone activity. All elements overlap, (i.e. to provide services, governance, human resources, finances, and supplies are needed. This section provides detail on each of the six building blocks, with examples from Afghanistan and other post-conflict environments.

Health leadership and governance

This is the most crucial but perhaps most complex component of any health system. Leadership is particularly important in transitional settings, as good leaders are also change agents – influencing those around them to adopt new practices. Health governance involves the sustainable delivery of health services of sufficient quality and equitability. Key components of effective health leadership and governance include policy guidance, health sector information provision and oversight, collaboration and coalition-building, regulation, system design, and accountability (WHO, 2007b).

Weak leadership and poor governance are defining characteristics of fragile states. Health regulation and oversight in a weak and possibly corrupt system are not effective. It is therefore imperative that international engagement in post-conflict reconstruction is focused on building or repairing the relationship between state and society, through (i) *supporting state legitimacy and accountability* by addressing democratic governance, human rights, civil society engagement, and peace-building, and (ii) *strengthening the capacity of state institutions to fulfil their core functions.* Efforts to strengthen health systems should address policies, information provision and oversight, collaboration, regulation, system design, and accountability, with clear indicators and targets established to measure their attainment. WHO has developed a toolkit to assist this process (WHO, 2008a).

Health ministries in post-conflict states can face considerable challenges in tracking the activities of the numerous health organizations that may operate independently, each with different goals, reporting requirements, time-frames and funding sources. To strengthen state managerial capacity, health actors can engage in planning with ministries to ensure that their goals, activities, reporting and timing align with government plans and priorities. Donors and NSPs can work with MoH staff in shared planning processes and focus their resources and activities on areas in which the MoH requires support. Mechanisms that support such approaches include sharing office space within the MoH and regularly exchanging ideas in targeted coordination meetings. For example, in Afghanistan, during early reconstruction, NSP staff, technical consultants and donors assisted the Ministry of Public Health (MoPH) with development of policies and medium-term expenditure frameworks for an equitable standardized package of health services to ensure the best results with available resources. Coordination was especially effective in the early transition period, when enthusiasm and support were high. Nearly a decade later, and with a technically competent staff in place, the MoPH is facing the challenge of sustaining sufficient levels of external commitment.

Health financing

Most health systems involve a mix of public and private financing and provision. Prepayment mechanisms such as taxation and health insurance are generally non-existent in post-conflict countries. Poor populations with a high burden of disease are therefore greatly reliant on private sector health services. Out-of-pocket payments contribute to financial shocks often culminating in an endemic cycle of poverty and ill-health. For many in post-conflict states, the only way to access essential health care is via services that are free at the point of care.

In early recovery settings, MoHs may struggle to establish and maintain effective health financing mechanisms. During the transition from relief to development, the mix and sequencing of aid can create funding gaps. The present use of aid mechanisms is often reactive, and reduction or withdrawal of humanitarian funding can result in the contraction of health services during sometimes long delays before adequate development funding begins. This is partly due to the need to develop or strengthen the MoH and departments. As MoHs are not always in a position to take on direct service provision, mechanisms have been developed to engage many of the NSPs that provided health services during conflict. Mechanisms include contracting out of services and private-to-public transition models (Canavan et al., 2008).

Contracting out, first piloted in Haiti and Cambodia in the 1990s, involves a competitive bidding process and selection of NGO and agency subcontractors based on quality and cost criteria. For example, after the war in Liberia ended in 2003, Liberia chose to tackle health sector challenges by using contracting to: (i) increase and sustain access to a basic package of health services (BPHS); (ii) provide support for improving the quality of service provision; (iii) leverage partner capacity until the county health teams could resume management of health facilities and the workforce. Liberia's Ministry of Health and Social Welfare (MoHSW) has worked with partners to stand-ardize the contracting model, increasing cohesive implementation of the National Health Plan. Additionally, MoHSW established the health sector pool fund, using national capacity and internal management, which donors use to finance the National Health Plan and minimize the efforts required for donor reporting and compliance.

Health service delivery

Health service delivery is the most visible part of a health system and represents the final output of the other five health system building blocks. Service delivery in fragile contexts is increasingly through packages of esssential health services, partly as it tends to facilitate donor funding and partly to support rapid scale-up of essential health services. Afghanistan, South Sudan, Liberia, and DRC have established packages that define and guide service delivery.

The Afghanistan BPHS, initiated in 2003 and last revised in 2010, covers priority health concerns in Afghanistan (e.g. maternal and newborn health, child health and immunization, public nutrition, infectious diseases, mental health, disability, essential drugs). The BPHS is offered at seven types of health facilities, ranging from community health workers to district hospitals. In 2005, the MoPH introduced an additional essen-tial package of hospital services defining service delivery at provincial and referral hospitals. Both packages have helped standardize service delivery, facilitated donor funding, and strengthened monitoring and evaluation.

Medical supplies and vaccines

Pharmaceuticals are essential to health systems and account for about 30% of total health expenditure in developing countries. Building effective and accountable national procurement and management systems is gaining recognition on the health system strengthening agenda. Nevertheless, in post-conflict reconstruction when governance is still weak, regulation of the supply and quality of medical products is often equally weak. With the high burden of disease contributing to a high demand for medications, the lack of effective regulatory mechanisms, trained staff, and testing equipment makes these countries inevitable 'dumping grounds' for unwanted, poor-quality or fake medicines.

Humanitarian supply chains tend to be highly fragmented, with each agency respon-sible for its own logistics supply cycles, training and guidelines. As contracting out of health services to NGOs gains popularity, this fragmentation will likely continue to exist unless MoHs actively pursue the establishment of a transparent and reliable centralized system to reduce costs and improve efficiency. Centralized procurement, supply, storage and distribution systems have often ceased to function, and where they do, they often lack resources and are vulnerable to corruption. Financial hardships, coupled with the collapse of these procurement and supply chains, could provide impetus for governments in post-conflict and fragile states to introduce large-scale, competitive purchasing of effective, low-cost generic drugs, but supporting this kind of activity is rarely a donor priority. Advocacy and coordination around a centralized, regulated procurement systems should be a key activity in post-conflict health system strengthening.

Government drug supply chains are organized on the basis of procurement units, central stores, transport, and dispersed storage or distribution centres. Whether this distribution chain delivers acceptable drugs to end users depends on different parameters, including funding, payment discipline, integrity (e.g. absence of fraud, theft, corruption), storage and transportation infrastructure, human resources, procurement capacity, planning, inventory management, and quality assurance. As implied by the term 'supply chain', the weakest link will define overall performance.

The development and support of relevant policies could improve coordination, effectiveness, and regulation of the supply of drugs, vaccines and medical materials. In some post-conflict settings, government regulation exists only on paper or can be highly corrupt or ineffective. In Afghanistan, contracting out has led to the need for most NGOs to procure their own drugs and medical supplies. International NGOs generally work with international tenders, while local NGOs work with local supply companies. Imported drugs are subject to control and clearance by customs and the MoH. Lack of warehousing capacity at the airport and borders means that drugs can be stored in the hot sun or freezing cold for months before clearance is granted, reducing the quality of drugs purchased. Delays often result in drug stock-outs, leaving agencies to purchases from local, largely unregulated markets. Insecurity and theft hinder transport, with some trucks simply 'disappearing' on the road.

Human resources

The health workforce is the most costly resource of any MoH, yet may receive the least attention or funding. In many post-conflict countries, much of the health workforce has left the country or moved to the cities due to the limited number of professional opportunities available to them. This results in shortages and imbalances in the distribution of remaining workers. Deteriorating capacities of accredited training institutions have often led to the development cadres of health staff whose competence for safe practice is not easily demonstrable. After prolonged periods of instability, capacity-building and in-service training programmes need to consider that significant gaps exist in levels of knowledge transmitted through primary, secondary and professional education.

In the rush to scale up health service delivery during reconstruction, there is a tendency to conduct ad hoc health worker training to address urgent short-term needs, while structural support of development and implementation of national workforce policies and investment plans may not be prioritized by either governments or donors. It does not necessarily have to be this way. For example, in Afghanistan health actors demonstrated the need to create a new cadre of health professional, community midwives, to address the country's high maternal mortality rates. This initiative was supported by government, donors, NGOs and communities.

In health facilities across post-conflict states, workers struggle to do their jobs in less than ideal conditions. How can capacity and motivation be rebuilt or created in a manner that avoids dependency and promotes sustainability? Investment in human resources is crucial to the success of health service delivery. An ideal workforce has sufficient competent, fairly distributed, responsive and productive staff. Limited health budgets and human resources in post-conflict states restrict governments' ability to achieve these targets. Where staff are available, training is often outdated or of poor quality, and training and hiring health workers and managers at all levels is a considerable challenge. However, there may be local resources available that are easily overlooked because they are not part of the health system (e.g. refugees or internally displaced persons with adequate training, NGO staff) who can contribute to government capacity-building without adding significant financial or training burdens to the health system. In Afghanistan's BPHS, three distinct forms of capacity development are identifiable: (i) on-the-job capacity development such as skills training and retraining for health staff; (ii) training in supervision skills, especially for those supervising community health workers; and (iii) facility management training for those responsible for management of facilities.

Information systems

Regardless of contextual differences, all post-conflict states require support in the establishment and strengthening of health information and surveillance systems, development of standardized data collection and analysis tools, and regular collation and dissemination of health statistics. Donor funding is conditional upon demonstrable progress and impact, while planning requires a body of data to facilitate evidence-based decision-making.

A well-functioning health management information system (HMIS) ensures the production, analysis, dissemination and use of reliable and timely information on health determinants (e.g. prevalence of risk factors, availability of services), health system performance, and health status. Monitoring and reporting at national and international levels require regular effective sub-national data collection. In fragile settings, where routine monitoring information may be unavailable or inconsistent, health information often relies on ad hoc surveys. Census data tend to be incomplete or severely outdated, as significant population movement can make these data unreliable. However, where systems are transparent and externally verified, they can minimize corruption and waste.

Although challenging, a good HMIS is achievable in fragile contexts, but will require considerable technical support, capacity-building and time. Supporting health information systems requires establishing a common set of essential indicators and data collection mechanisms that reflect national health priorities and capacity. It should include data, disaggregated by gender, age, and location where appropriate, on the following:

- birth and death registration;
- coverage indicators;
- facility-based data on access and coverage of key interventions;
- financial expenditure.

Tools and guidelines geared towards strengthening national health information systems have been developed by a consortium of partners (WHO/HMN, 2008).

✏️ **Activity 13.2**

Consider a post-conflict context with which you are familiar. Using the information provided in the discussion above, describe the major constraints being faced in strengthening the health system in your country of choice.

Monitoring and evaluating health system strengthening

WHO has produced an operational framework on monitoring and evaluation of health systems strengthening, which also applies to post-conflict and fragile states (WHO, 2010b). The related matrix in Figure 13.2 indicates how health inputs are reflected in outputs, outcomes and impact for the six health system building blocks. System inputs, processes and outputs reflect health system capacity, while outcomes and impact reflect health system performance. An effective monitoring and evaluation system should measure changes in health system inputs (e.g. human and financial resources) and outputs (e.g. levels and distribution of health service access). Results, such as equity, coverage of key interventions, and improved health levels, can then be captured by the system.

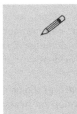

Activity 13.3

New models of service delivery in post-conflict settings, focused on non-state providers, have emerged in recent years.

13.3.1 What trade-offs may be necessary?
13.3.2 How should governments work towards monitoring, regulating or strengthening non-state providers?

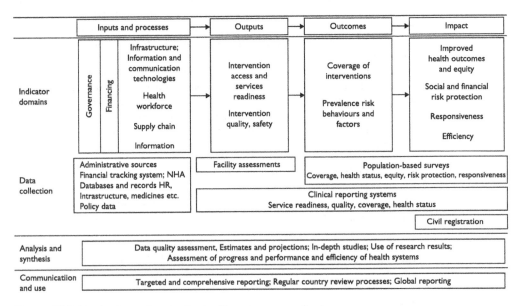

Figure 13.2 Monitoring and evaluating health system strengthening

Source: WHO (2010b).

Conclusions

This chapter shows that health system strengthening is a complex, context-specific process that needs to address all the independent building blocks. A range of humanitarian and development actors, including national and sub-national government, donors, NSPs and local communities, work on specific and often overlapping tasks in the rebuilding of health services disrupted by conflict. New service provision initiatives, such as contracting out, appear initially positive but more information is needed. The next chapter considers issues related to the health system in state-building and peace-building.

Feedback on activities

Feedback on Activity 13.1

13.1.1 Though each country context is different, the longer the state has experienced conflict and poor governance, the more disrupted the health system will generally be. Public institutions generally change slowly, and some staff may stay in the hope of reward once a functional government is in place. However, infrastructure deteriorates significantly as qualified health staff leave the country.

13.1.2 At times conflict is focalized and does not affect the entire country. For example, in Nepal the government health facilities continued running, but government supervision was not possible as rebels were barring access. Infrastructure that was poor pre-conflict cannot deteriorate much further, even during periods of fragility.

Feedback on Activity 13.2

In many post-conflict countries, major constraints are: (i) weak leadership and a poorly regulated health sector, both public and private, (ii) insufficient funding, (iii) poor-quality medical supplies and regular stock-outs, (iv) lack of qualified staff, with those available often poorly trained, and (v) lack of reliable data on disease burden, service delivery, population size, numbers and types of human resources, all leading to a lack of accessible and quality health services. This could be due in part to conflict or insecurity, lack of resources, and a lack of interest by the international community. In some countries, financial resources may be available, but the country does not have adequate human resources and infrastructure to absorb and make use of these funds.

Feedback on Activity 13.3

13.3.1 A number of trade-offs may be necessary between delivering health services through NSPs and strengthening health systems. Key elements to consider are:
- speed of delivery versus quality of the process;
- delivering health services in response to local needs versus emphasizing capacity-building;
- establishing long-term institutions versus temporary structures for project implementation;
- scaling up rapidly while still maintaining an intensive focus on governance and sustainability;

- bypassing local authority structures in favour of streamlined implementation mechanisms – at the risk of longer-term resentment and weakened sense of ownership.

13.3.2 Service delivery through NSPs appears a way forward for health sectors in many post-conflict states. However, it requires clear policy approaches (e.g. contracting out essential health packages) and a functional monitoring and evaluation system to ensure that service delivery is of adequate quality and effective. Initial results suggest that government-based service delivery may be less expensive, but also of poorer quality. However, competition among NSPs for Afghan health sector contracts may have contributed to lower bids for BPHS delivery than actually needed to provide quality health services. Combined with significant public sector corruption, this is a worrying development that could have detrimental effects on the health system. Regulation and strong monitoring and supervision systems for NSPs may be preferable to government-run service delivery, but data to support this are still lacking.

Health in state-building and peace-building 14

Egbert Sondorp, Annemarie ter Veen and Natasha Howard

Overview

The aim of this chapter is to provide an overview of state fragility and introduce the potential contribution of health system strengthening and health service provision to **state-building** and peace-building. Concepts from the global health policy and security literature will be used to explore these relatively new concepts for public health practitioners.

Learning outcomes

After completing this chapter, you should be able to:

- describe state fragility, including its importance for health systems
- discuss current debates on the role of health system strengthening in state-building and peace-building
- consider the role of health in combined approaches to state-building and peace-building

State fragility

Defining fragility

The concept of state fragility, originating in political science, has become increasingly important in global health policy and health security discourses. States and contexts are considered fragile when state structures lack the legitimacy or effectiveness to provide for basic development, security and human rights of their populations. Fragility may be characterized by weak governance, instability, persistent extreme poverty or inequity, lack of territorial control, frequent or persistent conflict, external shocks, and lack of either will or ability to provide basic services, including health services (Bertocchi, 2010; Moreno-Torres and Vallings, 2005).

Conceptual typologies of fragility

Donor agencies have classified state fragility into varying typologies according to context, three of which are outlined below. The first, developed for DFID, describes three types of political weakness (Moreno-Torres and Anderson, 2004): (i) *weak but willing,* in which government capacity is an obstacle to policy implementation; (ii) *strong but unresponsive,* in which state capacity is directed to achieving development goals but may not be inclusive or equitable; (iii) *weak-weak,* in which both state capacity and political will are lacking. The second, developed for the World Bank, divides states into four categories: (i) prolonged crisis or impasse; (ii) post-conflict or political transition; (iii) gradual improvement; and (iv) deteriorating governance (World Bank, 2005). This overlaps somewhat with the third typology, currently used by USAID (Table 14.1), which lists four possible conditions for fragility, based on the primary components of state legitimacy and state effectiveness (Newbrander, 2006). *Legitimacy* (i.e. willingness or political will) is defined as the ability of government to work in the public interest and demonstrate fairness to all groups when providing security and services. *Effectiveness* is defined as the capacity of government to (i) maintain security and order and (ii) provide public goods and services to citizens.

Regardless of typology, it may be inappropriate to categorize a whole country as a fragile state. Some areas may be stable and relatively peaceful, transitioning to post-conflict, while active conflict is confined to specific areas (i.e. deteriorating governance in pockets or regions). China and India, both large and very diverse countries, are good examples of this.

Drivers and measurement of state fragility

Drivers of fragility are often circular and self-reinforcing (e.g. instability increases poverty, which increases conflict and thus increases instability). Weak institutions and population income levels are both considered major drivers and often also consequences of fragility (Bertocchi, 2010; Moreno-Torres and Vallings, 2005).

The most widely used fragility index is arguably the World Bank's Country Policy and Institutional Assessment (CPIA). It rates country policies and institutions on a scale from 1 to 6, against four clusters of criteria: (i) economic management; (ii) structural

Table 14.1 Characteristics of state fragility

	Deteriorating governance	Arrested development	Post-conflict transition	Early recovery
Effectiveness (capacity)	• declining	• low, for extended periods	• low, but ready to rise	• increasing
Legitimacy (will)	• declining	• low, for extended periods	• transitory	• increasing
Manifestations and risks of fragility	• increasing risk of violence	• chronic underperformance • potential for violent responses to government failures	• recent violence and potential for relapses • humanitarian crisis	• potential funding gaps, as humanitarian aid declines and development funding may not have started

Source: Adapted from Newbrander (2006).

policies; (iii) policies for social inclusion and equity; and (iv) public sector management and institutions. For example, fragility may be categorized as scoring 3.2 or below (e.g. World Bank) or scoring in the bottom two quintiles (e.g. OECD/DAC). However, these scores are criticized for equating underdevelopment with fragility.

Other indices include the Country Indicators for Foreign Policy (CIFP) fragility index, which measures weaknesses in three fundamental dimensions (authority, legitimacy, capacity); the Failed States Index, based on 12 vulnerability indicators; and the Index of State Weakness in the Developing World, which provides an aggregate rating of 20 economic, political, security and social welfare indicators.

Fragility and health

What is evident from each of the fragility typologies outlined is that categorization as a fragile state or context is generally based on the relationship between governmental *will* and *capacity* to provide key public services. When either government will or capacity is weakened, health systems cannot function optimally.

Post-conflict terminology does not necessarily fit fragile states, as state fragility can be a threat to post-conflict recovery. While some states can progress from conflict towards peace and stability, others regress into further instability. Thus, not all conflict-affected states are at a recognizable stage along the humanitarian to state-building continuum outlined in Figure 12.1, and rebuilding health systems can be particularly challenging.

Humanitarian responses are the primary means of health sector support in contexts of deteriorating governance, arrested development, and the early stages of post-conflict transition. However, they are not designed for long-term support, while development assistance normally requires greater stability than found in fragile contexts. The potential threat of a fragile or 'failing' state creates mutual interest among both global development and security communities in workable solutions. Major donors that have increasingly engaged with fragile states include the World Bank, DFID, and OECD/DAC.

Activity 14.1

Make a list of 10–12 countries you would consider to be fragile states. Using the USAID typology, classify these countries into four categories according to what you know about their current political context.

Concepts of state-building and peace-building

Defining state-building

State-building is defined as constructing or reconstructing governance institutions capable of providing physical and economic security to residents of the country. It is the process by which states enhance their ability to function and involves supporting the development of internal governance processes of a state to enhance political stability and economic viability (Whaites, 2008).

The role of health systems in state-building

Effective health system strengthening contributes to state-building. The OECD lists state-building, in its third principle of engagement, as the central objective of international engagement in fragile states and says that the building of effective, legitimate and resilient states should be the common goal of all parties (OECD/DAC, 2007). Both humanitarian and health development donors have identified the health system as an important institution of state legitimacy, and several arguments have been forwarded for health system and service delivery strengthening in support of state-building.

It has been hypothesized that an inverse relationship exists between the health service needs of a population and the expectations that government will ensure service availability. Healthier populations with access to sophisticated health systems are seen to have higher expectations than poor populations with high disease burdens. This leads to the additional hypothesis that populations will appreciate services if they are offered, and importantly appreciate the provider. This hypothesis underpins much of the health service provision in 'hearts and minds' counterinsurgency operations (Thompson, 2008). It also underpins the idea that health services provided, or at least organized, by the government will contribute to increased state legitimacy in post-conflict situations (Rubenstein, 2009).

There is insufficient evidence yet whether government provision of health services strengthens or weakens state legitimacy. An argument in favour of service delivery enhancing legitimacy is the popularity of insurgency groups such as Hezbollah and Frelimo, with their emphasis on basic service delivery (OECD, 2008). Evidence from Iraq suggests that service provision through relatively small rapidly executable projects, which meet immediate local needs, enhances relations with local communities (Mashatt et al., 2008). However, Wilder found the opposite in Afghanistan, due to unmet or zero-sum community expectations, inappropriate projects, broken promises and corruption (Wilder, 2009).

This apparent contradiction may have much to do with the way services are provided, particularly issues such as to whom services are provided, by whom, by what financial means and through which accountability mechanisms. Donors may influence public expectations by enabling citizens to voice their demands (e.g. by promoting participatory approaches to defining needs, setting high quality standards, accountability mechanisms and transparency), although the extent to which aid instruments shape the nature of public expectations is not yet clear (Baudienville, 2010).

The social contract concept of health as a public good, while not technically correct in economic terms, has gained popular support as an advocacy tool (Smith and MacKellar, 2007). Advocates argue that if health care is provided free at point of use, based on need rather than ability to pay, this can legitimize increased tax collection and thus build government legitimacy. Again, evidence remains inconclusive.

Another argument for state-building through health suggests that as health-sector strengthening requires strengthening health governance, by doing so it contributes to state-building in the health sector (Eldon et al., 2008). However, Eldon et al. concluded that the impact of health sector interventions on wider state-building remains unclear, and called for further research on the potential for strengthening the state–society compact through decentralized bottom-up approaches.

Activity 14.2

Consider the countries you included in the list you drew up in Activity 14.1.

14.2.1 Did each country you selected fit neatly into a particular category?
14.2.2 Do you think any would have been classified in another category five or ten years ago, and if so, what changed this?

Defining peace-building

Peace-building is designed to prevent the start or resumption of violent conflict, creating a sustainable peace through activities addressing potential root causes of conflict and creating societal expectations of peaceful conflict resolution and stability. In 2007, the UN Secretary-General's Policy Committee agreed that peace-building strategies should (i) be coherent, tailored and based on national ownership, and (ii) comprise carefully prioritized, sequenced, and therefore relatively narrow sets of activities.

The role of health services in peace-building

Several arguments support the role of health system strengthening in peace-building. The 'Health as a Bridge for Peace' framework, accepted by the 51st World Health Assembly in 1998, draws on human rights, medical ethics, and humanitarian principles. The notion that health can provide a neutral space in which reconciliation and peace-building may be fostered is demonstrated at the simplest level in negotiated 'days of tranquillity' to allow vaccination campaigns. Common terminology, related to the Bridge for Peace concept, describes improved health services as part of the 'peace dividend', aiding further stabilization and peace-building.

An economic argument that improved health may contribute to improved wealth and therefore be a detriment to renewed conflict, takes the association between poverty and conflict into account. The reverse argument, that ill-health contributes to conflict, has been used to justify improved services in fragile contexts.

The emergence of epidemics is of particular concern among health security advocates. For example, high HIV prevalence countries could destabilize or even collapse, while newly emerging diseases such as severe acute respiratory syndrome (SARS) and avian influenza could threaten regional conflict (Brown, 2011).

A final argument is that conflicts may lead to widespread mental disorders, which in turn become a barrier to reconciliation and peace-building in post-conflict states. As with state-building, while the arguments are emotive, the capacity for health improvements to strengthen peace-building remains unclear (De Jong, 2010).

Activity 14.3

Discuss how health system strengthening might promote peace-building in a post-conflict country of your choice.

Future directions

Integrating state-building and peace-building approaches

Haider argues that state-building seeks to transform states and make them more responsive, while peace-building seeks to transform societal relationships. She describes how bottom-up peace-building approaches have focused on conflict prevention, diplomacy and local capacities for peace, but underemphasized institutional strengthening. Top-down state-building approaches have focused on stabilization, security and central government institutions, but underemphasized civil society, inclusivity and relationship-building (Haider, 2012).

Demonstrated inadequacies with both civil society peace-building approaches and institutional state-building approaches have led to increasing convergence of the concepts among policy-makers. Key areas for convergence, highlighted by DFID and OECD, include: analysing causes of conflict and fragility; supporting inclusive political settlements; promoting peaceful dispute resolution mechanisms; developing core state functions; responding to public expectations; and strengthening state–society relations, citizenship and sociopolitical cohesion (Haider, 2012).

The role of health and health care in these integrated approaches has yet to be determined. However, there is considerable scope for health policy-makers, researchers, and practitioners to develop these concepts further.

Strengthening the evidence base

There is insufficient evidence to conclude whether improved health systems and service delivery contribute significantly to state-building and peace-building, or whether different health institution-building or delivery methods would impact differently on these processes.

Over several decades, the humanitarian community has developed and tested models of health planning, implementation, monitoring and evaluation, largely resulting in effective, evidence-based approaches to addressing health in conflict-affected contexts. Approaches to fragility and post-conflict recovery are still fairly new, but an increasing number of humanitarian and development actors are exploring synergies between these sectors and how both can play a role in transition, recovery, state-building and peace-building processes. This provides hope that, despite the obvious challenges, these processes will benefit from accumulating research and experience over the coming years.

Conclusions

Conceptual frameworks for the link between health and fragility and health and state-building have emerged (Eldon et al., 2008; Kruk et al., 2010) and a next step is to strengthen the evidence base on the role of health in state-building and peace-building. This is the final topical chapter. The next chapter provides a concluding summary.

Feedback on activities

Feedback on Activity 14.1

The matrix below provides an example of countries you may have included

Fragility typology (feedback)

Deteriorating governance	Arrested development	Post-conflict transition	Early recovery
Syria	North Korea	Afghanistan	Rwanda
DRC	Guinea	Liberia	Cambodia
Somalia		Libya	Nepal

Feedback on Activity 14.2

14.2.1 Countries seldom fit neatly into categories. Somalia, listed in Activity 14.1 under 'deteriorating governance', is often classified as a 'failed state' – governance in certain parts of this country is non-existent and cannot really deteriorate further. Afghanistan is listed under post-conflict transition, but could also be listed under 'deteriorating governance' as state legitimacy appears to be decreasing and there is an increasing risk of violence throughout the country.

14.2.2 Some countries have undergone rapid or slow changes. Syria was considered a stable country only very recently, but governance in certain parts of the country has deteriorated significantly, triggering a humanitarian crisis. Libya is in a similar situation – the civil conflict in 2011 lasted a short time, but moved it from an oppressive regime to one that is currently being rebuilt. South Sudan has gone through several transitions – the signing of the Comprehensive Peace Agreement and installation of the autonomous government of Southern Sudan ended the civil war in 2005, and it became an independent country in 2011.

Feedback on Activity 14.3

Peace-building emphasizes bottom-up local-to-global thinking, relationship-building, inclusiveness, community empowerment, and non-violent conflict resolution. Health system strengthening is usually approached via top-down state-building approaches. You might have discussed strengthening community-level health services, community referral mechanisms, local health governance committees, or strengthening relationships and communication between providers and communities.

Conflict and health concepts and priorities

Natasha Howard

Overview

The aim of this concluding chapter is to apply concepts from preceding chapters to broader policy debates and highlight priorities for further study.

Learning outcomes

After completing this chapter you should be able to:

- identify concepts and issues from the humanitarian context, health interventions, and reconstruction efforts
- relate these concepts to broad priorities, including the nature of humanitarian engagement in a globalized world

Concepts and issues in conflict and health

Context

Conflict, in the form of collective political violence, affects millions of people globally. Yet current analysis indicates a major decline in the number and deadliness of global conflicts (Human Security Report Project, 2011). Some potential reasons for this decline include the changes in the global security environment (e.g. greater state and non-state engagement in global governance and interstate issues), development and the demographic transition (e.g. increased socioeconomic development in many countries and regions), and fewer battle deaths due to the changing nature of warfare technology. The result has been that civil and terrorist conflicts now lead research and policy agendas.

Global conflict issues are increasingly recognized. Global-local effects are particularly noticeable in the increased profile of *columbite-tantalite*, tin, and other conflict minerals (e.g. conflict diamonds are addressed in UN General Assembly Resolution A/RES/55/56). Warfare technology has changed tremendously, increasing asymmetrical and unconventional conflicts in which belligerents may never see each other and 'soft' (i.e. more accessible) non-combatants may be targeted. The aim of this concluding chapter is to apply concepts from preceding chapters to broader policy debates and highlight priorities for further study.

Three main approaches have informed analysis of conflict. Realist approaches focus on increasing global governance, including increasing professionalism of the humanitarian sector. Liberal approaches focus on increasing democratization and global economic interdependence. Constructivist approaches focus on changing global norms and the reduced acceptability of conflict and violence.

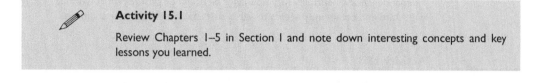

Activity 15.1

Review Chapters 1–5 in Section 1 and note down interesting concepts and key lessons you learned.

Humanitarian health interventions

Humanitarian health interventions, from needs assessment to service delivery and evaluation, have become increasingly professionalized, coordinated and complex.

Coordination and accountability have received considerable attention. The consolidated appeals process and cluster approach are relatively new initiatives to coordinate action and reduce gaps and overlap in service provision. Good donorship principles encourage communication between donors to achieve similar purposes. Joint needs assessments and evaluations are increasingly common. These initiatives are responses to perceived needs among humanitarian actors at a global level, and are unlikely to disappear even though they may be significantly revised in the coming years.

Security and protection of both beneficiaries and staff have become more complex and agency-dependent as conflict has changed. Humanitarian workers are expected to be aware of their rights and obligations within international humanitarian and human rights legal frameworks.

The epidemiological transition from infectious 'diseases of poverty' to 'diseases of wealth', combined with experiences from the AIDS pandemic, has increased interest in the sustainability of humanitarian programming efforts. For example, how can the support of patients, started on antiretrovirals or other long-term medications, be handed over to effective health care services once humanitarian providers have left? How can overarching issues, such as gender equity, disability or inclusion, be appropriately supported by humanitarian health workers?

Activity 15.2

Review Chapters 6–11 in Section II and note down interesting concepts and key lessons you learned.

Reconstruction

Debates about sustainability, whether and how best to address the handover of facilities and programmes, and growing recognition of the need to strengthen and support vulnerable fragile states, have influenced humanitarian engagement in post-conflict reconstruction. Humanitarian engagement has traditionally focused on **acute emergency** and **post-acute emergency phases**. Early recovery, peace-building and state-building are relatively new areas of work for the humanitarian sector. Action within these spheres has required new ways of operating, including active creation or strengthening of working relationships with development sector actors.

Humanitarian principles and short-term (e.g. immediate live-saving) methods of engagement are less effective in stabilization and recovery/development. For example, independence and neutrality may no longer be useful or positive when working closely with state and community actors towards sustainable development solutions.

Activity 15.3

Review Chapters 12–14 in Section III and note down interesting concepts and key lessons you learned.

Concepts and broader priorities

Policy debates

Health is a basic human right and involves more than reduced mortality and morbidity. Violent armed conflict is, by definition, dangerous for human health and it can be argued that efforts to reduce conflict will have a positive effect on health and other human development indicators.

A number of key policy debates are ongoing within the humanitarian sector. These include the nature of humanitarianism, the transition from relief to development, the role of coordination, and how to strengthen evaluation and improve quality. These relate to broader human security debates, including the following:

* What is causing the falling trend in excess mortality in conflict-affected countries (e.g. data collection issues, choice of baseline, actual reductions)?
* Can development be a long-term form of conflict prevention (e.g. does socio-economic development drive reductions in conflict, or is it a consequence)?
* What are the likely effects of increased UN-led initiatives to reduce and manage conflict (e.g. increasing coordination, accountability and professionalization among both humanitarian and security actors)?
* How will humanitarianism and health interventions evolve, given the changing nature of conflict and evolving aid architecture?

Evidence and research

It is likely that many humanitarian health initiatives will continue to improve over time, as 'best practice' and/or 'lessons learned' exercises continue to be incorporated into policy-making and programme implementation. For example, evidence is currently needed on the influence of differing methods of health reconstruction, the inclusiveness of health policy setting, and community involvement in planning and implementation, on the outcomes of post-conflict recovery processes.

While humanitarian providers are generally best situated to determine priorities and ask the questions, they can usually benefit from external technical support from the private sector or academia in conducting operational and more in-depth research.

Collaboration

Collaboration, dialogue and teamwork, in support of conflict-affected populations, are both useful and frustrating. For humanitarian health actors, collaboration is increasingly multi-sectoral and multidisciplinary.

Multi-sectoral collaboration has been discussed throughout this book, particularly in connection with other sectors within the humanitarian system (e.g. shelter, protection, water, sanitation, and hygiene). Collaboration with the development sector has become increasingly important as the humanitarian remit extends to health system strengthening and reconstruction. Collaboration, or at least dialogue, with the security sector may also be increasingly important.

The humanitarian sector has always been multidisciplinary. However, the need for technical support as interventions become more complex has led to a number of ongoing collaborations between humanitarian and academic actors. This has brought another kind of multidisciplinarity to humanitarian work, as epidemiologists, anthropologists and policy analysts add their perspectives. An example of these partnerships is the Reproductive Health Access, Information and Services in Emergencies (RAISE) initiative, developed by the Mailman School of Public Health at Columbia University and Marie Stopes International. Others began as academic projects and developed charitable status. Two examples are Jhpiego, now an NGO but originally founded as the Johns Hopkins Program for International Education in Gynecology and Obstetrics, and the Malaria Consortium, originally part of the London School of Hygiene & Tropical Medicine.

Conclusions

This chapter has highlighted some issues for further consideration, future research and strengthened collaboration. Humanitarian health action and conflict and health as a multidisciplinary area of study have changed tremendously in past decades. We hope this introductory book provides a foundation from which to continue in this important field.

Feedback on activities

Activity 15.1

You may have listed some of the following:

Chapter 1	• the shift to globalized 'network wars' and non-state combatants
	• political and economic explanatory theories of conflict
Chapter 2	• the cost of conflict and indirect effects of conflict on societies
	• vulnerability and resilience
Chapter 3	• health risk factors and consequences of conflict
	• epidemiological assessment (e.g. CMR, U5MR, excess mortality)
Chapter 4	• the main actors and approaches in international conflict responses
	• how health fits into the broader response
Chapter 5	• the origins and structure of the humanitarian system
	• the humanitarian principles

Activity 15.2

You may have listed some of the following:

Chapter 6 • humanitarian health assessment types and approaches
• data collection needs (e.g. demographics, health status, systems) and methods

Chapter 7 • right-to-health concepts
• humanitarian health service delivery approaches

Chapter 8 • greatest burden infectious diseases in conflict-affected settings
• infectious disease risk assessment

Chapter 9 • the increasing importance of chronic diseases and SRH among conflict-affected populations and availability of comprehensive SRH guidance
• need for specialist nutrition assessment and management

Chapter 10 • using the logframe approach in conflict-affected settings
• evaluation types and approaches

Chapter 11 • protection strategies and legal obligations
• the security triangle

Activity 15.3

You may have listed some of the following:

Chapter 12 • differences between transition, early recovery and recovery
• the analytical framework for health sector recovery

Chapter 13 • actors in health system strengthening
• the WHO health system building blocks

Chapter 14 • conceptualizing state fragility
• differences between state-building and peace-building

Glossary

Acute emergency phase This phase begins immediately after the impact of the disaster and may last for up to three months. It is characterized by initial chaos and a high crude mortality rate (CMR). It ends when daily CMR drops below 1 per 10,000 population.

Anthropometric This describes the measurement of individuals, in humanitarian field surveys, to determine the height and weight of children in order to identify the proportion of the population suffering from acute malnutrition.

Assessment A process of collecting and analysing context-specific information to determine population resources, capacities, needs, and threats at a single point in time.

Case fatality rate The number of deaths from a certain disease out of the number of cases of that disease.

Chronic emergencies These are protracted, complex situations, sometimes called 'complex emergencies', characterized by extreme vulnerability and displaying a combination of: (i) weak or hostile governance, (ii) political oppression or armed conflict, (iii) population displacement, (iv) poor health and social indicators, including excess mortality, and (v) minimal international interest or funding.

Chronic infectious disease These include such diseases as tuberculosis and HIV that are communicable but can be managed for several years with the proper drug regimen.

Civil war This usually takes place within the borders of a country.

Clean delivery kit To reduce infection during home births, most contain a bar of soap for hand-washing, a plastic sheet for the delivery surface, a new razor blade for umbilical cord cutting, clean string for cord tying, and pictorial instructions on delivery and hand-washing.

Cluster In the context of humanitarian reform, a cluster is a group of agencies, organizations and/or institutions interconnected by their respective mandates, which works together towards common objectives. The purpose of the cluster is to foster timeliness, effectiveness and predictability while improving accountability and leadership.

Cluster approach A mechanism for sector coordination introduced by the UN in December 2005 to enhance the ability of humanitarian coordinators to manage humanitarian responses effectively.

Cold chain A popular term for a temperature-controlled supply chain required for many biologicals (e.g. vaccines) from manufacture to shipping, warehousing, storage, and administration.

Community-based management of severe malnutrition This consists of four core components: (i) community outreach, (ii) outpatient care for children under age 5 with severe acute malnutrition (SAM) without complications, (iii) inpatient care for SAM with complications, and (iv) supplementary feeding for the management of moderate acute malnutrition, offered in the context of broader preventive services.

Community-based organization (CBO) A civil society non-profit organization, usually operating within a single local community.

Community-based rehabilitation (CBR) Initiated in the mid-1980s, this has evolved into a multi-sectoral strategy to empower persons with disabilities to access and benefit from education, employment, health and social services.

Complex emergencies *See* **chronic emergencies**.

Conflict-affected A set of conflict-affected states was derived for each year between 1999 and 2009 using the Uppsala Conflict Data Programme's (UCDP) database to determine the incidence of active conflict in a given year, both with and without state actor involvement, and involving more than 25 battle deaths annually.

Cost of conflict This is defined as a measure of welfare loss between the current situation in a country and the welfare that the country would have achieved in the absence of conflict.

Crude mortality rate (CMR) This is the key public health indicator for monitoring crises, estimating the death rate in a population (e.g. number of deaths per 10,000 population per day), unadjusted for age or sex.

Direct effects of conflict These are normally attributable to combat (e.g. combat-related deaths and injuries).

Disability This describes one or more conditions (e.g. physical, cognitive, mental, sensory, emotional, developmental) limiting a person's movements, senses, or activities.

Disabled people's organizations These are set up, run and controlled by disabled people and focus on human rights and equality for disabled people.

Disease When the invasion of the body by a pathogen manifests outward symptoms and signs.

Disease surveillance A structured, routine, regular system of collecting, analysing, and interpreting health data to monitor trends and inform disease prevention and control programmes.

Displaced persons These individuals leave their homes, usually in groups and with an intention to return, due to significant perceived danger (e.g. natural disaster, threat, violent conflict).

Early recovery This process applies development principles to humanitarian situations, to stabilize national and sub-national capacities from further deterioration so they can provide a foundation for full recovery.

Emergency threshold Mortality rate above which an emergency considered to be occurring, it is usually taken as a crude mortality rate of 1 per 10,000 population per day or as an under-5 mortality rate of 2 per 10,000 population per day.

Endemic A disease that occurs normally in a particular area, throughout the year or with seasonal peaks.

Epidemic An increase in incidence of a disease more than is expected for the specific population and time of year.

Epidemiological triad A standard model of infectious disease causation, including (i) an external agent, (ii) a susceptible host, and (iii) an environment that brings host and agent together so that disease can occur.

Epidemiology The study of the distribution and determinants of health states or events in specified populations, and the application of this study to the control of health problems.

Essential health services These are preventive and curative health services that address the health needs of a population and prevent and reduce excess morbidity and mortality. In conflict situations services will include interventions for communicable as well as non-communicable diseases, child health, sexual and reproductive health, injury and mental health.

Ethnicity A social grouping based on common consciousness of shared origins and traditions.

Ethnic conflict A conflict between ethnic groups or where ethnic difference is central to the conflict.

EWARN This is an early warning system for infectious diseases surveillance, initiated by WHO and generally based on clinical description, with the main aim of detecting epidemics.

Excess mortality Deaths above what would be expected based on the non-crisis mortality rate in the population of interest (i.e. observed mortality rate minus expected non-crisis mortality rate × population at risk × time-period of interest); this quantifies mortality attributable to the crisis, expressed as a rate or as a total number of excess deaths.

Faecal-oral transmission This occurs through consumption of food or drink that has been contaminated with faeces, either through faeces contaminating water sources or hands, and then contaminating water, feeding children, eating or preparing food.

Food security This includes both physical and economic access to food that meets dietary needs and food preferences. It is built on three pillars: (i) food availability, i.e. having sufficient quantities of food available on a consistent basis; (ii) food access, i.e. having sufficient resources to obtain appropriate foods for a nutritious diet; (iii) food use, i.e. appropriate use based on knowledge of basic nutrition, care, water and sanitation.

Forced displacement This refers to the situation of persons who are forced to leave their homes due to conflict, violence, persecution or human rights violations.

Fragile state/country This is defined principally as a fundamentally inadequate government that is unable to perform the functions necessary to meet citizens' basic needs and expectations in poverty reduction, development and safeguarding the security and human rights of populations.

Gender The social differences between females and males that are learned, changeable, and widely varying both within and between cultures.

Gender-based violence (GBV) Any physical, sexual, psychological, economic or socio-cultural harm resulting from power imbalances that exploit distinctions between males and females that may be perpetrated in private or public settings.

Global acute malnutrition (GAM) This is measured as the index of weight for height among children aged 6–59 months, which reflects recent weight loss or gain, as a proxy health indicator for the whole population. GAM is calculated as a Z-score, defined as a weight-for-height index less than −2 standard deviations from the mean weight of a reference population of children of the same height and/or having oedema. Z-scores measure the divergence of an individual experimental result from the mean, assuming the sampling distribution is normal, and transform it into a standard normal distribution. Commonly used thresholds for GAM are: < 5% = acceptable, 5–9.9% = poor, 10–14.9% = serious, > 15% = critical. Population nutritional status is a basic indicator, with CMR, to assess the severity of a humanitarian crisis. GAM of more than 10% generally identifies an emergency.

Golden hour The initial minutes to hours where immediate medical intervention is most likely to preserve life in trauma patients.

Greed This is considered a cause of conflict based on a desire similar to crime but on a larger scale.

Green war hypothesis The hypothesis that environmental change and degradation can be a source of poverty and insecurity and thus of conflict.

Grievance This is a motivation based on a sense of injustice in the way a social group is treated, often with a strong historical dimension.

Health service delivery This involves provision of promotive, preventive and curative services to ensure health within the population. Good health services are those that deliver effective, safe, and quality care to those who need it, when needed, in an efficient way.

Health system All the organizations, institutions, resources, and people whose primary purpose is to improve health. As part of early recovery efforts, the international community often works to reconstruct and rebuild the capacity of health systems.

Health system strengthening This requires building capacity in critical components of health systems (whether within and between the different building blocks such as human resources or financing, or at or between different levels such as local or national level), to achieve more equitable and sustained improvements across health services and health outcomes.

Health system strengthening building blocks These include (i) leadership, governance and (ii) financing of health systems, as well as the strengthening of (iii) health information, (iv) service delivery, (v) human resources, and (vi) medical and drug supply systems.

Healthy life year (HLY) A structural indicator that provides an estimate of expected remaining years lived from a particular age without long-term activity limitation.

Hearts and minds agenda This amorphous agenda is common in military humanitarian assistance, often including one or more objectives: (i) to provide a tactical entry point into communities that are potentially hostile to military interests; (ii) to allow the military to build connections, influence local perceptions, and acquire knowledge; (iii) to address underlying causes of violent extremism through alleviating poverty.

Herd immunity Immunity that occurs when an entire population or group of animals or people is no longer affected by a particular infection, such as through universal vaccination.

Honour killing A murder, usually committed by male family member(s) against a female family member, to avenge a perceived dishonour brought upon the family.

Host community The population into which a displaced population of refuges or internally displaced persons settles, either in segregated camps or a dispersed manner.

Human resource development (HRD) Adequately trained and supported health workers are the cornerstone of health care delivery systems, influencing access, quality and costs of health care and effective delivery of interventions for improved health outcomes, including progress towards the achievement of the health Millennium Development Goals and Health for All.

Humanitarian action This covers actions relating to the relief of human suffering, especially when there is an actual or imminent threat to life, health, subsistence or security. Actions are generally in response to an acute crisis and characterized by relatively short time-frames and goals.

Humanitarian actor Those involved in the humanitarian service sector (e.g. NGOs, UN, donors), providing relief in emergencies and protracted displacement. Generally, members of the military are not considered humanitarian actors.

Humanitarian assistance Aid to an affected population that complies with the basic humanitarian principles and falls within three categories, based on degree of contact: (i) direct assistance is face-to-face distribution of goods and services; (ii) indirect assistance is at least one step removed from affected populations (e.g. transporting relief goods or personnel); (iii) infrastructure support involves providing general services, such as road repair or power generation that facilitate relief, but are not necessarily visible or solely to benefit the affected population.

Humanitarian emergency This can be broadly categorized into conflict, natural disaster, and food insecurity.

Humanitarian imperative The belief that action should be taken to prevent or alleviate human suffering arising from disaster or conflict whatever the circumstances. This principle is paramount.

Humanitarian norms *See* **humanitarian principles**.

Humanitarian placebo A situation in which humanitarian assistance is provided to civilian populations in place of a broader political strategy that addresses root causes of the conflict.

Humanitarian principles Four main principles (i.e. humanity, impartiality, independence, and neutrality) provide the foundations for humanitarian action. They are considered central to ensuring access to affected populations in a range of humanitarian contexts including natural disaster, conflict or complex political emergency. Organizations and individuals operating as humanitarian actors will be working to these principles in some form.

Humanitarian system This is the large diverse collective of institutions, organizations and actors involved in humanitarian action.

Humanity This is one of the four core humanitarian principles, and states that all human beings are born free and equal in dignity and rights leading to the humanitarian imperative. The objective of humanitarian action is to protect life and health, ensure respect for human beings, and address human suffering wherever it is found.

Immunization campaign The international community organizes immunization days in conflict-affected states, often negotiating ceasefires with warring groups to access and vaccinate as many people as necessary to achieve population immunity. Measles and polio are two common vaccines delivered in conflict-affected areas.

Impartiality One of the four core humanitarian principles, this states that humanitarian assistance must be provided solely on the basis of need, giving priority to the most urgent cases of distress and making no distinctions on the basis on nationality, ethnicity, gender, religious belief, class or political opinions.

Incidence The frequency of new cases in a specified population and specified time period (e.g. new disease cases per 10,000 population per week).

Independence Operational independence is one of the four core humanitarian principles, and states that humanitarian action must be autonomous from the political, economic, military or other objectives that any actor may hold with regard to areas where humanitarian action is being implemented.

Indicator A variable or combination of variables (qualitative or quantitative) used as a measure of a specific area of interest, such as health status of the population.

Indirect effects of conflict These do not immediately result from a physical or weapon attack but are due instead to a combination of conflict-related factors that often continue into the post-conflict period (e.g. poverty due to economic disruption, disease due to lack of treatment access).

International NGO *See* **non-governmental organization**.

Institutional actor In international relations, institutional actors are the agencies and institutions involved in the policy process. These are sometimes separated into traditional state and political institutional actors (e.g. parliaments, governments, judiciary, political parties) and extra-institutional actors (e.g. trade unions, constituted advisory bodies, business, interest groups, lobbies, influence networks, media, and criminal groups).

Integrated vector management This is a rational decision-making process to optimize use of resources for evidence-based vector control and target contextually appropriate measures, such as long-lasting insecticidal nets, indoor residual insecticide spraying, and larval source management.

Internally displaced persons (IDPs) Persons or groups who have been forced or obliged to flee or to leave their homes or places of habitual residence, particularly because of the effects of armed conflict, situations of generalized violence, violations of human rights or natural or human-made disaster, and who have not crossed an internationally recognized state border.

International conflict A conflict that occurs between two or more countries.

International donors The organizations, political owners, civil servant managers, sources, and uses of funds. They include supranational (e.g. the European Commission), multilateral (UN system agencies, World Bank), and bilateral (e.g. AusAID, CIDA, DFID, SIDA, USAID) agencies.

International humanitarian law (IHL) The set of rules that govern the protection of persons who are not, or no longer, involved in violent conflict and the means and methods by which war is conducted.

Law of war *See* **international humanitarian law**.

Livelihood How people routinely earn money to meet basic family needs. Its loss can be devastating for conflict-affected households.

Logical framework (logframe) This analytical tool, originally developed by the US Department of Defence, is a 4 × 4 matrix showing goals, objectives, activities, and intended outcomes that is often used to plan, monitor, and evaluate projects.

Malnutrition This condition results from an unbalanced diet in which certain nutrients are lacking, excessive, or in the wrong proportions (e.g. global acute malnutrition, global chronic malnutrition, micronutrient malnutrition).

Medical model of disability A model by which illness or disability results from a physical condition intrinsic to the individual, may reduce quality of life, and causes disadvantages.

Minimum Initial Service Package (MISP) A package of guidance and activities that is intended to support provision and planning of essential sexual and reproductive health services in acute and post-acute crises.

Mid-upper arm circumference (MUAC) Measured at the mid-point between the tip of the shoulder and the tip of the elbow on the left arm, and useful for assessing nutritional status in children.

Mixed migration The complex cross-border population movements related to safeguarding physical and economic security and can include refugees, asylum seekers, and economic and other migrants.

Morbidity The burden of illness or disease in a population.

Mortality The burden of death in a population.

Mortality rate The number of deaths in a specified population and time period. *See also* **crude mortality rate, under-5 mortality rate**.

Negotiated access Traditionally access to non-combatant populations was agreed between warring parties. The rise of armed non-state actors increased direct informal access agreements between non-state humanitarian agencies and armed actors. Since the 'War on Terror', non-state combatants have increasingly regarded humanitarian actors as viable targets and thus undermining any negotiation.

Neutrality This is one of the four core humanitarian principles, and states that humanitarian actors must not take sides in hostilities or engage in controversies of a political, racial, religious or ideological nature.

New wars Often civil wars of low-intensity conflict, involving multiple local and global actors, in which the distinction between war and organized crime is blurred.

Non-governmental organization (NGO) This is a legally-constituted association, operating independently of governments, with a social or sociopolitical agenda, and not conventionally for profit.

Non-state actors In international relations terms, these are organizations with sufficient power to influence and cause change in politics that are not state structures or established state institutions (e.g. they have no legal sovereignty or legal control over a country or its citizens). Such actors include multinational corporations, media, NGOs, armed groups, and criminal gangs.

Nutritional rehabilitation (NGO) This is a supervised process of inpatient or community-based supplementation of macro- and micronutrients to bring malnourished patients back to a state of nutritional well-being.

Old wars Ideological wars between nation-states, fought by armed forces in uniform, where decisive encounters occurred on the battlefield.

Pathogen A bacteria, virus, or parasite that has the ability to infect and cause disease in a person.

Peace-building A range of measures targeted to reduce the risk of lapsing or relapsing into conflict, to strengthen national capacities at all levels for conflict management, and to lay the foundations for sustainable peace and development.

Post-acute emergency phase This usually begins when daily CMR drops below 1 per 10,000 population.

Post-conflict The phase of recuperation, peace-building and reconstruction following a conflict, often with the presence of a multilateral peace-keeping mission and no recurrence of violence in the past year.

Prevalence The frequency of existing cases in a defined population at a particular point in time (point prevalence), or over a given period of time (period prevalence), as a proportion of the total population.

Project cycle This is a multi-stage conceptual process that every project or programme goes through. Usual categories are (i) identification/inception, (ii) preparation, (iii) appraisal, (iv) implementation and monitoring, (v) completion, (vi) evaluation.

Protracted conflict A term sometimes used in international relations to describe complex or chronic emergencies.

Rate A ratio in which the denominator is expressed in units of person-time at risk.

Ready-to-use therapeutic food This includes brands such as Plumpy'nut or BP-100, which are lipid-based, resistant to contamination, have an extended shelf-life without refrigeration or need for preparation, and do not require medical oversight during administration.

Recidivism When applied to conflict-affected or fragile states, this means the high proportion of states where conflict reignites after a peace agreement is reached.

Refugee The 1951 Convention Relating to the Status of Refugees defines a refugee as someone who, owing to a well-founded fear of being persecuted for reasons of race, religion, nationality, membership of a particular social group or political opinion, is outside the country of his nationality, and is unable to or, owing to such fear, is unwilling to avail himself of the protection of that country.

Resilience This theory incorporates concepts of psychological and community resilience theories to explain the ability of an individual, community or society to adapt to and recover from the effects of major hazards, such as conflict.

Resource curse This refers to the hypothesis that countries and areas with abundant natural resources, specifically non-renewable resources (e.g. minerals, oil), tend to have worse development outcomes than countries with fewer natural resources.

Responsibility to Protect This is an internationally recognized norm that highlights the responsibility of states to protect their citizens from grave violations of human rights, such as genocide and other crimes against humanity. If the state cannot protect its citizens, or if the state is the actor perpetrating these crimes, then the international community has the responsibility to intervene to stop these crimes.

Risk factor Patient characteristic (either inherited, such as a blood group, or behavioural, such as smoking and diet habits) or environmental factors (such as exposure to conflict) associated with an increased or decreased probability (risk) of developing disease or other outcome.

Rule of law This holds when individuals and government submit to and are regulated by national and international laws rather than the arbitrary action of an individual or group.

Severe acute malnutrition (SAM) This is defined as a Z-score below −3 standard deviations from, or less than 70% of, the mean weight-for-height among children in the WHO reference population, by visible severe wasting, or by the presence of nutritional oedema.

Sexual violence Any non-consensual sexual action, including rape, attempted rape, sexual exploitation and sexual abuse; it is considered a sub-category of gender-based violence.

Social contract This philosophical hypothesis, initially promoted by Thomas Hobbes (1651), John Locke (1689), and Jean-Jacques Rousseau (1762), to explain the appropriate relationship between government and individuals; is used by modern theorists such as Pettit to explain potential causes of civil conflict.

Social vulnerability This is the susceptibility of an individual or community to negative effects from a hazard (e.g. abuse, conflict).

State In international relations terms, this refers to an autonomous political unit with defined physical boundaries and government system (also called a country, nation or nation-state). State also refers to the executive, legislative and the judiciary branches of central governments.

Standard precautions Designed to prevent transmission of blood-borne diseases and pathogens (e.g. HIV, hepatitis B) when health care is provided by treating human blood, body fluids, tissues, and cells as infected.

State-building This is the process by which states enhance their ability to function, through constructing or reconstructing governance institutions capable of providing physical and economic security to residents of the country.

Transition The period between immediate aftermath of crisis and either recovery (i.e. restoration of pre-crisis conditions) or development (i.e. improvement to a satisfactory level beyond pre-crisis conditions).

Transition funding gap During the post-conflict transition, the limited humanitarian health services that exist often come under threat of contraction. This is caused by a reduction in humanitarian funding for health combined with a slow inflow of development aid.

Transitional settlement This is intended to provide temporary shelter in cases of conflict or natural disaster, and ranges from emergency responses to durable solutions.

Triage The process of distinguishing acute cases needing referral to hospitals from cases requiring immediate medical attention and those that can wait for medical care.

Triage sieve An initial, rapid assessment to establish priority of treatment and evacuation.

Triage sort A more detailed and accurate assessment based on wider physiological parameters.

Uncompensated incident A disaster or catastrophe where all existing resources are overwhelmed requiring external assistance.

Under-5 mortality rate (U5MR) This is a key indicator to monitor the health status of children in crises settings, and is the number of deaths among children 0–59 months old among the total population of children 0–59 months old in a specified time period (e.g. number of deaths per 10,000 population per day). Note that this is different from the standard demographic U5MR, which is the probability of dying before age 5 expressed per 1,000 live births.

Vector-borne disease A disease in which the pathogen is transmitted by way of an intermediate organism. The pathogen either requires the vector for part of its life cycle (snail) or requires the vector to penetrate human tissue (e.g. bite of mosquito, flea) so the pathogen can be passed into the human.

Vulnerable group A population group that would be vulnerable under any circumstances, due to physical or socioeconomic factors (e.g. young children).

Vulnerability *See* **social vulnerability**.

References

ACP (2011) *Secondary Data Review: Côte d'Ivoire* (third update). Geneva: Assessment Capacities Project.

Advanced Life Support Group (2002) *Major Incident Medical Management and Support: The Practical Approach in the Hospital*. London: BMJ Publishing Group.

ALNAP (2010) The role of national governments in international humanitarian response. 26th Annual Meeting 16–27 November, Kuala Lumpur.

Amnesty International (2004) Sudan: Darfur: Rape as a weapon of war: Sexual violence and its consequences. http://www.cmi.no/sudan/doc/?id=1082 [accessed 1 November 2011].

Anderson M (1999) *Do No Harm: How Aid Can Support Peace or War*. London: Lynne Rienner.

Bailey S (2010) Somalia food aid diversion. Overseas Development Institute – Feature. 16 March. http://www.devex.com/en/articles/somalia-food-aid-diversion [accessed 6 July 2012].

Bailey S and Pavanello S (2009) Untangling early recovery. HPG Policy Brief 38, Overseas Development Institute, London.

Ballentine K and Nitzchke H (2003) Beyond greed and grievance: Policy lessons from studies in the political economy of armed conflict. International Peace Academy Report.

Baudienville G (2010) Aid instruments in fragile and conflict-affected situations: Impacts on the state- and peace-building agenda. Overseas Development Institute, London.

Belton R (2009) Competing definitions of the rule of law: Implications for practitioners. Carnegie Endowment for International Peace.

Bertocchi G (2010) The empirical determinants of state fragility. University of Modena. http://www.voxeu.org/index.php?q=node/4833 [accessed 6 July 2012].

Binder A, Meier C and Steets J (2010) Humanitarian assistance: Truly universal? A mapping study of non-Western donors. GPPi Research Paper No. 12, Global Public Policy Institute, Berlin.

Bornemisza O, Ranson MK, Poletti TM and Sondorp E (2010) Promoting health equity in conflict-affected fragile states, *Social Science and Medicine*, 70, 80–8.

Borton J (2009) Future of the humanitarian system: Impacts of internal changes. John Borton Consulting, Berkhamsted.

Bozzoli C, Bruck T and Sottsas S (2010) A survey of the global economic costs of conflict, *Defence & Peace Economics*, 21, 165–76.

Brinkerhoff D (2008) From humanitarian and post-conflict assistance to health system strengthening in fragile states: Clarifying the transition and the role of NGOs. http://www.healthsystems2020.org/content/resource/detail/2153/ [accessed 9 July 2012].

Brown T (2011) 'Vulnerability is universal': considering the place of 'security' and 'vulnerability' within contemporary global health discourse, *Social Science and Medicine*, 72, 319–26.

Buhaug H and Lujala P (2004) Accounting for scale: Measuring geography in quantitative studies of civil war, *Political Geography*, 24, 399–418.

Canavan A, Vergeer P and Bornemisza O (2008) *Post-conflict Health Sectors: The Myth and Reality of Transitional Funding Gaps*. Commissioned by the Health and Fragile States Network. Amsterdam: Royal Tropical Institute.

Caulfield LE, de Onis M, Blossner M and Black RE (2004) Undernutrition as an underlying cause of child deaths associated with diarrhea, pneumonia, malaria, and measles, *American Journal of Clinicial Nutrition*, 80, 193–8.

Chan EY and Sondorp E (2007) Medical interventions following natural disasters: Missing out on chronic medical needs, *Asia-Pacific Journal of Public Health*, 19 (Spec. No.), 45–51.

Checchi F (2010) Estimating the number of civilian deaths from armed conflicts, *Lancet*, 375, 255–7.

Checchi F, Gayer M, Grais R and Mills E (2007) Public health in crisis-affected populations: A practical guide for decision-makers. HPN Network Paper 61, Overseas Development Institute, London.

Clark CJ, Everson-Rose SA, Suglia SF, Btoush R, Alonso A and Haj-Yahia MM (2010) Association between exposure to political violence and intimate-partner violence in the occupied Palestinian territory: A cross-sectional study, *Lancet*, 375, 310–16.

Coghlan B, Ngoy P, Mulumba F, Hardy C, Bemo VN, Stewart T, Lewis J and Brennan RJ (2009) Update on mortality in the Democratic Republic of Congo: Results from a third nationwide survey, *Disaster Medicine and Public Health Preparedness*, 3, 88–96.

Collier P (2000) Economic causes of civil conflict and their implications for policy, unpublished paper, Washington DC. World Bank.

Collier P (2008) *The Bottom Billion: Why the Poorest Countries are Failing and What Can Be Done about It*. Oxford: Oxford University Press.

Collier P and Hoeffler A (2004) Greed and grievance in civil war, *Oxford Economic Papers*, 56, 563–95.

Collier P, Hoeffler A and Rohner D (2009) Beyond greed and grievance: Feasibility and civil war, *Oxford Economic Papers*, 61, 1–27.

Connolly MA, Gayer M, Ryan MJ, Salama P, Spiegel P and Heymann DL (2004) Communicable diseases in complex emergencies: Impact and challenges, *Lancet*, 364, 1974–83.

Cramer C (2006) *Civil War Is Not a Stupid Thing: Accounting for Violence in Developing Countries*. London: C Hurst & Co.

Cutter S, Emrich T and Burton S (2008) Baseline Indicators for Disaster Resilient Communities. *CARRI Workshop*. Broomfield, CO.

Darcy J and Hofman C (2003) According to need? Needs assessment and decision-making in humanitarian response. HPG Report 15, Overseas Development Institute, London.

De Jong JT (2010) A public health framework to translate risk factors related to political violence and war into multi-level preventive interventions, *Social Science and Medicine*, 70, 71–9.

Degomme O and Guha-Sapir D (2010) Patterns of mortality rates in Darfur conflict, *Lancet*, 375, 294–300.

DFID (2011) *Humanitarian Emergency Response Review*. Chaired by Lord Ashdown, 28 March. http://www.dfid.gov.uk/Documents/publications1/HERR.pdf [accessed 21 May 2012].

Di John J (2008) Conceptualising the causes and consequences of failed states: A critical review of the literature. LSE Destin Working Paper 25 – Development as State-Making, London School of Economics.

Domres B, Koch M, Manger A and Becker HD (2001) Ethics and triage, *Prehospital and Disaster Medicine*, 16, 53–8.

Doran G (1981) There's a S.M.A.R.T. way to write management's goals and objectives, *Management Review*, 70, 35–36.

Doull L (2011) NGOs and the cluster approach: A worthwhile investment? *Health Exchange*, 7.

Driscoll P, Skinner D and Earlam R (2000) *ABC of Major Trauma*, 3rd edn. London: BMJ Publishing Group.

du Mortier S and Coninx R (2007) Mobile Health Units in emergency operations. A methodological approach (HPN Network Paper 60). Humanitarian Practice Network, Overseas Development Institute, London.

Duffield M (2001) *Global Governance and the New Wars: The Merging of Development and Security*. London: Zed Books.

EC, UNDG and World Bank (2008) Joint Declaration on Post Crisis Assessments and Recovery Planning. http://betterpeace.org/files/EC_UNDG_WB_Joint_Declaration_on_Post_Crisis_Assessments_and_Recovery_Planning_25_Sep_2008.pdf [accessed 9 July 2012].

ECLAC (2003) *Handbook for Estimating the Socioeconomic and Environmental Effects of Disasters*. Mexico City: Economic Commission for Latin America and the Caribbean http://www.gdrc.org/uem/disasters/disenvi/eclac-handbook.html [accessed 6 July 2012].

Egal F (2006) Nutrition in conflict situations, *British Journal of Nutrition*, 96(Suppl. 1), S17–19.

Egeland J, Harmer A and Stoddard A (2011) To stay and deliver: Good practice for humanitarians in complex security environments. Policy and Studies Series. UN Office for the Coordination of Humanitarian Affairs, New York.

Eldon J, Waddington C and Hadi Y (2008) Health system reconstruction: Can it contribute to state-building? Health and Fragile States Network, London.

Galtung J (1969) Violence, peace, and peace research, *Journal of Peace Research*, 6, 167–91.

GHD (2003) Principles and good practice of humanitarian donorship. Good Humanitarian Donorship, Geneva.

GHWA, WHO, IFRC, UNICEF and UNHCR (2011) Scaling-up the community-based health workforce for emergencies. Global Heath Workforce Alliance.

Glaser M (2003) Negotiated access: Humanitarian engagement with armed nonstate actors. Carr Center for Human Rights Policy.

Global Humanitarian Assistance (2010) *GHA Report 2010*. Wells, Somerset: Development Initiatives.

Global Humanitarian Assistance (2011) *GHA Report 2011*. Wells, Somerset: Development Initiatives.

Golaz A (2010) Challenges of healthcare provision to IDPs in non-camp settings: The 2009 IDP crisis in Pakistan. Paper presented at Geneva Health Forum: Globalization, Crisis and Health Systems: Confronting Regional Perspectives, 20 April.

Goldstein JS (2011) Think again: War, *Foreign Policy*, September/October.

Grais RF, Strebel P, Mala P, Watson J, Nandy R and Gayer M (2011) Measles vaccination in humanitarian emergencies: A review of recent practice, *Conflict and Health*, 5, 21.

Gurr T (1970) *Why Men Rebel*. Princeton, NJ: Princeton University Press.

Haider H (2012) Statebuilding and peacebuilding in situations of conflict and fragility: Topic guide supplement. Governance and Social Development Resource Centre.

Hallam A (1998) Evaluating humanitarian assistance programmes in complex emergencies. Good Practice Review No. 7, Overseas Development Institute, London.

Handrahan L (2004) Conflict, gender, ethnicity and post-conflict reconstruction, *Security Dialogue*, 35, 429–45.

Harvey P, Stoddard A, Harmer A and Taylor G (2011) *The State of the Humanitarian System: Assessing Performance and Progress. A Pilot Study*. London: ALNAP. http://www.alnap.org/pool/files/alnap-sohs-final.pdf [accessed 14 May 2012].

Homer-Dixon T (2001) *Environment, Scarcity, and Violence*. Princeton, NJ: Princeton University Press.

Human Security Report Project (2011) *Human Security Report 2009/2010: The Causes of Peace and the Shrinking Costs of War*. New York: Oxford University Press.

Humanitarian Accountability Partnership (2010) The 2010 HAP Standard in Accountability and Quality Management. HAP International, Geneva.

IASC (2007) *IASC Guidelines on Mental Health and Psychosocial Support in Emergency Settings*. Geneva: Inter-Agency Standing Committee.

IASC (2008) *Civil-Military Guidelines & Reference for Complex Emergencies*. New York: UN.

IASC (2009) *Health Cluster Guide*. Geneva: WHO.

IASC (2010a) *Handbook for RCs and HCs on Emergency Preparedness and Response*. Geneva: Inter-Agency Standing Committee.

IASC (2010b) Removing user fees for primary health care services during humanitarian crises. http://www.who.int/hac/global_health_cluster/about/policy_strategy/EN_final_position_paper_on_user_fees.pdf [accessed 6 July 2012].

IASC (2011a) *IASC Guidance on Coordinated Assessments in Humanitarian Emergencies*. Geneva: Inter-Agency Standing Committee.

IASC (2011b) *IASC Guidance Note on Working with National Authorities*. Geneva: Inter-Agency Standing Committee.

ICRC (2004) What is international humanitarian law? Advisory Service on International Humanitarian Law, ICRC, Geneva.

ICRC (2007) Women in war: A particularly vulnerable group? http://www.icrc.org/eng/resources/documents/misc/women-vulnerability-010307.htm [accessed 31 March 2012].

ICRC (2011) Health care in danger: Making the case. ICRC, Geneva.

IFRC and ICRC (1996) Annex VI: The Code of Conduct for the International Red Cross and Red Crescent Movement and NGOs in Disaster Relief, *International Review of the Red Cross, No. 310.*

Interagency Health Evaluation (2005) Liberia: Final report.

International Displacement Monitoring Centre (2010) Internal Displacement: Global overview of trends and developments in 2010. http://www.internal-displacement.org/publications/global-overview-2010.pdf [accessed 6 July 2012].

Jones L, Asare JB, El Masri M, Mohanraj A, Sherief H and Van Ommeren M (2009) Severe mental disorders in complex emergencies, *Lancet,* 374, 654–61.

Kaldor M (1999) *New and Old Wars: Organized Violence in a Global Era.* Oxford: Polity Press.

Kaldor M (2007) *Human Security: Reflections on Globalization and Intervention.* Oxford: Polity Press.

Kaplan R (1994) The coming anarchy, *Atlantic Monthly,* 273, 44–76.

Keen D (2008) *Complex Emergencies.* Cambridge: Polity.

Kett M and Van Ommeren M (2009) Disability, conflict, and emergencies, *Lancet,* 374, 1801–3.

Kolieb J and Tasheebeva A (2009) Working Paper 1. The six grave violations against children during armed conflict: the legal foundataion. Office of the Special Representative of the Secretary-General for Children and Armed Conflict.

Krug EG, Dahlberg LL, Mercy JA, Zwi AB and Lozano R (eds) (2002) *World Report on Violence and Health.* Geneva: World Health Organization.

Kruk ME, Freedman LP, Anglin GA and Waldman RJ (2010) Rebuilding health systems to improve health and promote statebuilding in post-conflict countries: a theoretical framework and research agenda, *Social Science and Medicine,* 70, 89–97.

Lang R, Kett M, Groce N and Trani J (2011) Disability, the capability approach and human rights: The next steps in disability studies and practice, *European Journal of Disability Research,* 5, 206–20.

Lavell A (2000) An approach to concept and definition in risk management terminology and practice (final draft). ERD-UNDP, Geneva.

Lehmann U and Sanders D (2007) Community health workers: What do we know about them? The State of the evidence on programmes, activities, costs an impact on health outcomes of using community health workers. WHO, Geneva.

Lund C, De Silva M, Plagerson S, Cooper S, Chisholm D, Das J, Knapp M. and Patel V (2011) Poverty and mental disorders: Breaking the cycle in low-income and middle-income countries, *Lancet,* 378, 1502–14.

Mamdani M (1996) *Citizen and Subject: Contemporary Africa and the Legacy of Late Colonialism.* Princeton, NJ: Princeton University Press.

Mashatt M, Long D, and Crum J (2008) *Conflict-Sensitive Approach to Infrastructure Development.* Washington, DC: US Institute of Peace.

Maxwell D, Bailey S, Harvey P, Walker P, Sharbatke-Church C and Savage P (2012) Preventing corruption in humanitarian assistance: Perceptions, gaps and challenges, *Disasters,* 36 (1), 140–60.

Medact (2004) Enduring effects of War: Health in Iraq 2004. Medact, London.

Médecins Sans Frontières (2006) *Rapid Health Assessment of Refugee or Displaced Populations.* Paris: Médecins Sans Frontières.

Miller KE and Rasmussen A (2010) War exposure, daily stressors, and mental health in conflict and post-conflict settings: Bridging the divide between trauma-focused and psychosocial frameworks, *Social Science and Medicine,* 70, 7–16.

Mont D and Loeb M (2008) *Disability, Conflict, and Emergencies.* Washington, DC: The World Bank and Centers for Disease Control and Prevention.

Moreno-Torres M and Anderson M (2004) Fragile states: Defining difficult environments for poverty reduction. DFID, London. http://www.gsdrc.org/go/display/document/legacyid/1343 [accessed 6 July 2012].

Moreno-Torres M and Vallings C (2005) Drivers of fragility: What makes states fragile? PRDE Working Paper 7. http://webarchive.nationalarchives.gov.uk/+/http://www.dfid.gov.uk/Documents/publications/fragile-states/drivers-fragility.pdf [accessed 6 July 2012].

Murray CJ, King G, Lopez AD, Tomijima N and Krug EG (2002) Armed conflict as a public health problem, *British Medical Journal*, 324, 346–9.

Nathan L (2005) The frightful inadequacy of most of the statistics: A critique of Collier and Hoeffler on the causes of civil war. Discussion Paper no. 11, Crisis States Development Research Centre.

Newbrander W (2006) Arrested development in fragile states: Opportunities and guidance for USAID health programming. Arlington, VA: Basic Support for Institutionalizing Child Survival (BASICS) for USAID.

NutritionWorks (2011) The Harmonised Training Package: Resource Material for Training on Nutrition in Emergencies, Version 2. Emergency Nutrition Network, Global Nutrition Cluster.

OCHA (2010) Humanitarian Principles. http://ochanet.unocha.org/p/Documents/111031_OOM%20-%20Humanitarian%20Principles.pdf [accessed 21 May 2012].

OECD (2008) *Service Delivery in Fragile Situations: Key Concepts, Findings and Lessons*. Paris: OECD.

OECD/DAC (2002) *Glossary of Key Terms in Evaluation and Results Based Management*. Paris: OECD. http://www.oecd.org/dataoecd/29/21/2754804.pdf [accessed 9 July 2012].

OECD/DAC (2007) Principles for good international engagement in fragile states and situations. OECD. http://www.oecd.org/dataoecd/61/45/38368714.pdf [accessed 6 July 2012].

OECD/INCAF (2010) Guidance on transition financing: building a better response (draft version, 27 October). International Network on Conflict and Fragility.

Pavignani E and Colombo S (2009) *Analysing Disrupted Health Sectors: A Modular Manual*. Geneva: World Health Organization. http://www.who.int/hac/techguidance/tools/disrupted_sectors/en/index.html [accessed 23 May 2012].

Perrin P (1996) *War and Public Health: Handbook on War and Public Health*. Geneva: ICRC.

Pettit P (1997) *Republicanism: A Theory of Freedom and Government*. Oxford: Clarendon Press.

Pinker S (2011) *The Better Angels of Our Nature: Why Violence Has Declined*. New York: Viking.

Potter C and Brough R (2004) Systemic capacity building: a hierarchy of needs, *Health Policy and Planning*, 19, 336–45.

Prince M, Patel V, Saxena S, Maj M, Maselko J, Phillips MR and Rahman A (2007) No health without mental health, *Lancet*, 370, 859–77.

Redmond AD, Mahoney PF, Ryan JM and Macnab C (2005) *ABC of Conflict and Disaster*. London: BMJ Publishing Group.

Reilly R (2008) *Disabilities among Refugees and Conflict-Affected Populations*. Women's Commission for Refugee Women and Children.

RHRC (2011) *Distance learning module for the Minimum Initial Service Package for Reproductive Health in Crisis Situations*. Reproductive Health Response in Crises Consortium. http://misp.rhrc.org/ [accessed 4 April 2012].

Roberts B, Patel P and McKee M (2012) Noncommunicable diseases and post-conflict countries, *Bulletin of the World Health Organization*, 90(1):2, 2A.

Robertson DW, Bedell R, Lavery JV and Upshur R (2002) What kind of evidence do we need to justify humanitarian medical aid? *Lancet*, 360, 330–3.

Rubenstein L (2009) *Post-Conflict Health Reconstruction: New Foundations for U.S. Policy*. Washington DC: US Institute of Peace.

Ryan J, Mahoney P and Greaves I (2002) *Conflict and Catastrophes Medicine: A Practical Guide*. New York: Springer.

Slaymaker T and Christiansen K (2005) Community-based approaches and service delivery: Issues and options in difficult environments and partnerships. Overseas Development Institute, London.

Slim H (1997) Doing the right thing: Relief agencies, moral dilemmas and responsibility in political emergencies and war, *Disasters*, 21, 244–57.

Slim H and Bonwick A (2005) *Protection: An ALNAP Guide for Humanitarian Agencies*. London: ALNAP.

Smith D (2004) *Trends and Causes of Armed Conflict*. Berlin: Berghof Research Center for Constructive Conflict Management.

Smith RD and MacKellar L (2007) Global public goods and the global health agenda: problems, priorities and potential, *Global Health*, 3, 9.

Sondorp E (ed.) (2011) *French and Anglo Saxon: A Different Ethical Perspective?* London: Hurst & Co.

Sondorp E and Patel P (2003) Climate change, conflict and health, *Transactions of the Royal Society of Tropical Medicine and Hygiene*, 97, 139–40.

Sphere (2011) *The Sphere Handbook: Humanitarian Charter and Minimum Standards in Humanitarian Response*. Sphere Project.

Spiegel PB and Salama P (2000) War and mortality in Kosovo, 1998–99: An epidemiological testimony, *Lancet*, 355, 2204–9.

Spiegel PB, Checchi F, Colombo S and Paik E (2010a) Health-care needs of people affected by conflict: Future trends and changing frameworks, *Lancet*, 375, 341–5.

Spiegel PB, Hering H, Paik E and Schilperoord M (2010b) Conflict-affected displaced persons need to benefit more from HIV and malaria national strategic plans and Global Fund grants, *Conflict and Health*, 4, 2.

Spiegel PB, Mills E, Joffres, MR and Anema A (2011) The imperative to respond with appropriate and timely interventions to mass rape in conflict-affected areas, *AIDS*, 25, 391.

Steets J, Grünewald F, Binder A, de Geoffroy V, Kauffmann D, Krüger S, Meier C and Sokpoh B (2010) Cluster Approach Evaluation 2: Synthesis report. Global Public Policy Initiative.

Stewart F (2002) Root causes of violent conflict in developing countries, *British Medical Journal*, 324, 342–5.

Stoddard A, Harmer A and Haver K (2006) Providing aid in insecure environments: trends in policy and operations. HPG Report 23, Overseas Development Institute, London.

Stoddard A, Harmer A and DiDomenico V (2009a) Private security contracting in humanitarian operations. HPG Policy Brief 33, Overseas Development Institute, London.

Stoddard A, Harmer A and DiDomenico V (2009b) Providing aid in insecure environments: 2009 update. HPG Policy Brief 34, Overseas Development Institute, London.

Terry F (2002) *Condemned to Repeat: The Paradox of Humanitarian Action*. New York: Cornell University Press.

Thompson D (2008) *The Role of Medical Diplomacy in Stabilizing Afghanistan*. Washington DC: National Defense University Center for Technology and National Security Policy.

Tol WA, Barbui C, Galappatti A, Silove D, Betancourt TS, Souza R, Golaz A and Van Ommeren M (2011) Mental health and psychosocial support in humanitarian settings: Linking practice and research, *Lancet*, 378, 1581–91.

UNDG (2008) Guidance and good practice note on transitional results frameworks and matrices. World Bank.

UNDG (2009) *PCNA Tool Kit*. World Bank. http://pcna.undg.org/index.php?option=com_docman&task=cat_view&gid=7&Itemid=4 [accessed 6 July 2012].

UNDP (2001) Annual Report of the Administrator for 2000. DP/2001/14.

UNDP (2008) Policy on early recovery. Bureau for Crisis Prevention and Recovery, UNDP.

UNDP, World Bank and UN Development Group (2004) Practical guide to multilateral needs assessments in post-conflict situations.

UNICEF (2012) Health in emergencies. http://www.unicef.org/health/index_emergencies.html [accessed 4 April 2012].

UNISDR (2004) *Living with Risk: A Global Review of Disaster Risk Reduction Initiatives*. Geneva: UN Publications.

UNISDR (2009) UN International Strategy for Disaster Reduction Terminology on Disaster Risk Reduction. http://www.unisdr.org/we/inform/terminology [accessed 6 July 2012].

Uppsala Universitet (2012) Uppsala Conflict Data Programme. http://www.ucdp.uu.se/gpdatabase/search.php [accessed 6 July 2012].

Van Ommeren M and Tol WA (2011) Assessing mental health and psychosocial needs and resources: Toolkit for major humanitarian crises (draft version). WHO, Geneva.

Ventevogel P, Pérez-Sales P, Férnandez Liria A and Baingana F (2011) Integration of mental health into existing systems of care during and after complex humanitarian emergencies: An introduction to a special issue, *Intervention*, 9.

Ventevogel P, van de Put W, Faiz H, van Mierlo B, Siddiqi M, et al. (2012) Improving Access to Mental Health Care and Psychosocial Support within a Fragile Context: A Case Study from Afghanistan, PLoS Med 9(5): e1001225. doi:10.1371/journal.pmed.1001225

Vitale T and Corsellis A (2005) Transitional settlement displaced populations. The Shelter Project, Oxfam.

Waldman R (2011) How can we improve disaster response? Reforming the reforms, *Health Exchange*, 7.

Walker P (2007) The origins, development and future of the international humanitarian system: Containment, compassion and crusades. ISA 49th Annual Convention, Bridging Multiple Divides.

Walker P and Maxwell D (2008) *Shaping the Humanitarian World*. Abingdon: Routledge.

Watts CH, Foss AM, Hossain M, Zimmerman C, Von Simson R and Klot J (2010) Sexual violence and conflict in Africa: Prevalence and potential impact on HIV incidence, *Sexually Transmitted Infections*, 86 (Suppl 3), iii93–99.

Wessells M and Van Ommeren M (2008) Developing inter-agency guidelines on mental health and psychosocial support in emergency settings, *Intervention*, 6 (3), 199–218.

Whaites A (2008) States in development: Understanding state-building. DFID Working Paper.

WHO (2007a) Communicable disease risk assessment: Protocol for humanitarian emergencies. WHO/CDS/NTD/DCE/2007.4, June. http://www.who.int/diseasecontrol_emergencies/guidelines/Com_dis_risk_ass_oct07.pdf [accessed 15 May 2012].

WHO (2007b) *Everybody's Business. Strengthening Health Systems to Improve Health Outcomes. WHO's Framework for Action.* Geneva: World Health Organization.

WHO (2008a) Measuring health systems strengthening and trends: A toolkit for countries. http://www.who.int/healthinfo/statistics/toolkit_hss/EN_PDF_Toolkit_HSS_Introduction.pdf [accessed 6 July 2012].

WHO (2008b) *Outbreak Communication Planning Guide*. Geneva: World Health Organization.

WHO (2009) Guidelines for trauma quality improvement programmes. http://www.who.int/violence_injury_prevention/services/traumacare/traumaguidelines/en/index.html [accessed 4 November 2011].

WHO (2010a) *mhGAP Intervention Guide for Mental, Neurological and Substance Use Disorders in Non-Specialized Health Settings.* Geneva: World Health Organization.

WHO (2010b) Monitoring and evaluation of health systems strengthening: an operational framework. http://www.who.int/healthinfo/HSS_MandE_framework_Oct_2010.pdf [accessed 6 July 2012].

WHO (2010c) *World Health Report 2010. Health System Financing: The Path to Universal Coverage.* Geneva: World Health Organization.

WHO (2011a) *The Humanitarian Emergency Settings Perceived Needs Scale (HESPER): Manual with Scale.* Geneva: World Health Organization.

WHO (2011b) The Libyan Arab Jamahiriya: Civil unrest. Public health risk assessment and interventions, WHO/HSE/GAR/DCE/2011.1. World Health Organization, Geneva.

WHO (2012) Health service delivery. http://www.who.int/healthsystems/topics/delivery/en/index.html [accessed 4 April 2012].

WHO/HAC (2010) Guidance for health sector assessment to support the post disaster recovery process (version 2.2). World Health Organization, Geneva.

WHO/HMN (2008) Assessing the National Health Information System: An assessment tool. WHO/Health Metrics Network. http://www.who.int/healthmetrics/tools/Version_4.00_Assessment_Tool3.pdf [accessed 6 July 2012].

WHO, ILO, UNESCO and IDDC (2010) Community-based Rehabilitation: CBR Guidelines. Geneva: World Health Organization.

Wilder A (2009) Losing hearts and minds in Afghanistan, in P Fitzgerald (ed.), *Afghanistan, 1979–2009: In the Grip of Conflict.* Washington, DC: Middle East Institute.

Wisner B, Blaikie P, Cannon T and Davis I (2004) *At Risk: Natural Hazards, People's Vulnerability, and Disasters.*
    London: Routledge.

World Bank (2004) The costs of corruption. http://web.worldbank.org/WBSITE/EXTERNAL/NEWS/0,,
    contentMDK:20190187~menuPK:34457~pagePK:34370~piPK:34424~theSitePK:4607,00.html
    [accessed 14 November 2011].

World Bank (2005) Fragile states – good practices in country assistance strategies. IDA/R2005–0252.
    Report No. 34790. Operations Policy and Country Services, World Bank, Washington, DC.

World Bank (2011) *Conflict, Security, and Development. World Bank Development Report 2011.* Washington,
    DC: World Bank.

Yao, M. (2004) UNDP World Bank training presentation, Geneva.

Young H and Jaspers S (2006) The meaning and measurement of acute malnutrition in emergencies: A
    primer for decision-makers. HPN Network Paper No 56, Overseas Development Institute, London.

Index

*The **McGraw·Hill** Companies*

What's new from Open University Press?

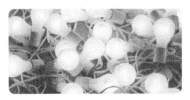
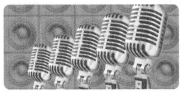

Education... Media, Film & Cultural Studies

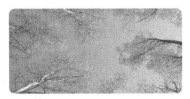
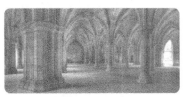

Health, Nursing & Social Welfare... Higher Education

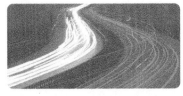
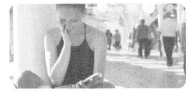

Psychology, Counselling & Psychotherapy... Study Skills

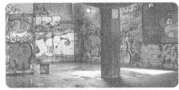

Keep up with what's buzzing
at Open University Press
by signing up to receive
regular title information at
www.openup.co.uk/elert

Sociology

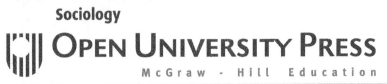

OPEN UNIVERSITY PRESS

McGraw - Hill Education